HAIR LOSS

Learn About Hair Loss Prevention Methods and
Regrowth Treatment

(The Ultimate Guide on Overcoming Postpartum
Hair Loss Depression for Human in Natural Ways)

Keith Jefferson

Published By Keith Jefferson

Keith Jefferson

Hair Loss: Learn About Hair Loss Prevention Methods and Regrowth Treatment (The Ultimate Guide on Overcoming Postpartum Hair Loss Depression for Human in Natural Ways)

ISBN 978-1-77485-397-9

Legal & Disclaimer

The information contained in this book is not designed to replace or take the place of any form of medicine or professional medical advice. The information in this book has been provided for educational and entertainment purposes only.

The information contained in this book has been compiled from sources deemed reliable, and it is accurate to the best of the Author's knowledge; however, the Author cannot guarantee its accuracy and validity and cannot be held liable for any errors or omissions. Changes are periodically made to this book. You must consult your doctor or get professional medical advice before using any of the suggested remedies, techniques, or information in this book.

TABLE OF CONTENTS

Introduction

This book provides practical steps and methods for how to stop and treat hair loss. Whatever your age or gender hair loss could become an issue. Certain conditions can be temporary however, the majority of them could cause permanent hair loss. It is essential to understand the signs of it right away, what you can do to prevent it, and also how to manage it. Although there are males who are able to handle this more easily but children and women can't cope with it well. This causes them to be stressed more mentally and emotionally which can affect their self-esteem. This is especially true for children younger than them, as some may be being bullied or anxious about the things that are happening to them.

Children also suffer from hair loss and its effects can be detrimental not only physically, but as well emotionally. Should you be a parent of children who suffer from this issue This book is ideal for you. This book will help you recognize the first indication of hair loss and stop it from happening. For women This book will make you aware about the devastation that many women do to their hair to look prettier. Some of these may result in permanent loss of hair which is devastating.

The loss of hair is also the result of an illness. This book is designed to aid you in determining hair loss that occurs in the early stages of health ailments you weren't aware of prior to. There are also certain medications that can trigger hair loss. This book can aid you through these stages , or to find ways to encourage healthy hair at this time.

In this book, you'll be able to understand the reasons behind hair loss, the causes and preventive measures that will aid in maintaining healthier hair. The book also provides solutions for both natural and medical. The book also covers ways to cause damage to your hair follicles and cause hair loss. These include the incorrect method of styling, the right treatments and even the nutrients that you must consume to encourage healthier growth of your hair.

This book will help you to get better hair and a better overall health…

Thank you so much for reading this book. I hope that you will enjoy it!

Chapter 1: The Reasons for hair loss

and damage

Most people lose approximately 40-60 hairs a day, up to 100 hairs every day. If you notice hairs falling off the brush or as you comb your hair, don't be discouraged instantly. If the amount of hair visible on your hairbrush is roughly the same, then there's usually no reason to be concerned. However, if it appears at all to you like the rate of loss is increasing, you should consider trying some preventative measures.

To be able to take the right measures to prevent hair loss you must determine the root of the issue.

The primary causes of baldness as well as substantial loss of hair are the following causes:

Health issues. Chronic diseases are often the cause of hair loss. Anemia, thyroid problems as well as stomach ailments, pneumonia and stomach problems can affect the health of hair loss. It's crucial to avoid delay consulting a doctor to get a diagnosis.

Stress. Continuous stress at work and family problems as well as other emotional issues cause us to be stressed and unbalanced. Stress isn't the only cause of hair loss it may also function as the primary reason behind problems related to a lack of volume, shine and a decrease in energy. Intense emotional experiences disrupt peripheral circulation. In the result, hair cells don't get enough nutrients and can fall out. Stress can cause hereditary hair loss.

Dieting too much and insufficient nutrition. The long-term adherence to strict diets and poor nutrition could put the body in danger due to the deficiency of vitamins needed to maintain the development and maintenance of hair.

The use of styling products for styling. The continuous and excessive use of mousses, sprays, hair coloring along with hairdryers and styling irons results in hair loss and eventually to loss of hair.

The incorrect use of hair care products. A lack of purification may cause hair follicles to become blocked and the pores of the scalp. This is why hair loss and fragility, along with the itching and hair loss.

Insufficient immunity. If your immunity is weak our bodies are particularly susceptible frequently to infections as well as chronic illnesses that in turn can hamper the health of hair.

Infections. In some instances hair loss is one of the most significant problems following an illness caused by fever and inflammation that trigger loss of hydration to the hair follicles.

Dandruff. The Trichologists (hair and scalp experts in hair and scalp) claim that dandruff is the main reason for hair loss. Dandruff can weaken the roots of hair and blocks the pores on the scalp. Whatever the reason for hair loss, it's important to combat this issue by using special shampoos, balsams, or antifungal medicines.

The use of medication. Certain medications contain ingredients which can build up in the body, negatively affecting the health and growth of hair.

Heredity. Unfortunately, the risk of hair loss and baldness usually passed down through the generations. If you're a victim of a family history of loss of hair don't put off visiting a doctor who treats trichology.

Hormonal imbalance. Alopecia androgenetica (baldness) may develop as you age due to an increase in sensitiveness of the follicles to the effects of dihydrotestosterone, a hormone. Through the action on this enzyme (5-alpha-reductase) testosterone is transformed into dihydrotestosterone. This causes the breakdown of proteins. Hair follicles aren't properly fed cease to function, shrink in size, and eventually die.

Pregnancy. Loss of hair is common due to hormonal changes. It's only temporary and therefore you don't have to take anything extra. It's enough to take care of yourself since this condition is likely to disappear within a few months.

Rapid changes in temperature. To safeguard your hair during the winter months, ensure that you wear an insulated hat and during summer, shield your hair from direct sunlight by making use of scarves and hats.

Environmental hazards. A higher risk of exposure to radiation, polluted water and air is a fact that cannot be escaped especially in big cities. All of these elements affect our health and deteriorate our hair health. A drastic change in our environmental conditions is usually the main reason behind severe hair loss.

Insufficient vitamins and microelements. In general, a diet that is not balanced is the reason for a variety of diseases. Hair loss is a common occurrence due to the fact that our bodies are deficient in vitamins. It is important to remember that alcohol and smoking can cause the destruction of all beneficial elements in our body. When vitamin deficiencies are present it is essential to take vitamin complexes.

Hair Types How to Determine Your Hair Type

It's crucial to know the kind of hair you have before you can begin to care for your hair in a proper manner. Hair is classified into hard and soft thin and thick curly, straight, curly and curly, dark and light healthy and damaged. But the most crucial aspect of appropriate care is to classify it by oiliness. Hair is classified based on the level of oiliness in normal, dry, and mixed hair kinds. The degree of oiliness in hair is dependent on the kind of skin. If you are aware of the kind of skin that you're dealing with, it's simple to figure out the hair type you have.

Hair with oily hair. Sebaceous glands in the scalp are overactive this can cause hair to be often covered in oil and appears messy. Hair that is oily will have dull shine, fast adhesion, and a sensation of greasiness upon contact. If your hair becomes extremely greased within a few days, then you are an oily hair type.

Normal hair. If, after 2-4 days of you wash your hair it appears fresh, shines in the sunlight, isn't electric, and is easy to comb this means you are of normal hair.

Dry hair. It appears dry and brittle, it has split ends, gets tangled rapidly, and is difficult to comb. Dryness in hair that is excessive can result due to the ineffective work of sebaceous glands, or due to improper care for your hair. If your hair doesn't appear clean for a prolonged period (6 weeks or longer) Your hair type is dry.

Mixed hair type. If you have hair that is long generally, you have an mixed hair type. In this instance the greasiness glands are unable to supply lubrication across the entire length of hair. In particular, this type of hair has oily at the root and over dry split, tangled and split ends. The roots are already oily to the touch after a few days. At this time, the hair's roots appear shiny and shiny, while the ends appear dry. You have an unusual type of hair.

Your hair's oiliness isn't an indefinite characteristic. Rather, it may change with the influence of hormones changes, age-related changes, adjustments in your diet and your overall health. Be aware of this to modify your hair care. When there is any oiliness, hair will be well-groomed and gorgeous, if it is properly treated.

Chapter 2: A Complete

Understanding of Hair Loss

Hair in humans develops everywhere on the face except for toes as well as the fingers of our hands. However, the majority of hairs are so thin that they appear almost invisibly. The hair that grows on our skin is comprised of keratin, an amino acid that is created within the skin's outer layers. skin's hair follicles. The average adult hair is comprised of between 100,000 to 150,000 hairs. In all 90 percent of your hair grows at any given moment, or perhaps at different phases of its development. Each follicle has their own unique life cycle, which is typically influenced by illness and age, as well as a myriad of other elements.

The lifecycle can be broken down into three stages:

* Anagen: Anagen is the hair's active growth which lasts from 2 to 6 years.

* Catagen refers to the growth phase of hair that is transitional which lasts from 2 to 3 weeks.

* Telogen The period of rest that usually lasts between 2 and three months. At close of period the hair is shed and is replaced with new hair and the cycle of growth starts again.

The rate at which hair grows is reduced as you get older.

Like the name suggests, hair loss is losing hair in any body part typically, your head is the most affected in this process. It is sometimes called hair loss or alopecia. The severity of loss of hair is different from a single region to the entire body. The appearance of inflammation or scarring is generally not evident.

It is normal to lose between 100 and 100 strands of hair every day, so don't be worried if you spot some hairs that aren't within your hair brush. This isn't the type of hair loss is being discussed in this instance. However, if you're losing a significant quantity in hair (perhaps more than 100 strands you lose a day) in a way that is obvious or causes concern, this is the type of hair loss this book will examine.

Hair loss is divided into two categories: genetic and reactive.

" *Reactive " indicates that your loss of hair is due to the trigger.

* Genetic: If the loss of your hair isn't the result of a trigger, chances are that you're genetically predisposed to losing hair which means that you will see a gradual but progressive decrease in the amount of your hair. The hair follicles will gradually shrink and will produce shorter and smaller hairs as you go through each growth cycle.

Diagnosis

The doctor you see will conduct a physical examination on you and will inquire about the medical history of your family and your relatives prior to making the diagnosis. They may also run these tests

Blood test A blood test is extremely beneficial since it could aid in identifying the medical issues associated with hair loss.

Scalp biopsy - If the diagnosis is not clear the doctor will perform a scalp biopsy as it helps distinguish between non-scarring and scarring forms and hair loss. The doctor may scrape skin samples or collect a few hair samples, typically near the edges of the bald patches, to assess the hair's root. This can help determine if the loss of hair is the result of an infection

Test of Pull Tests are essential to evaluate the degree of hair loss on your scalp. loss and determines the level of the process of shedding. The doctor will remove numerous dozens of hairs on three distinct areas on your head. The doctor will take a count of the hairs extracted and then examine them with the microscope. In normal circumstances, with each pull, no less than 3 hairs in each area should be released. A pull is considered to be successful when at least 10 hairs are pulled out.

The pluck test is not to be confused with pull tests. The pluck test is pulling hair but "by the roots". The hair's root is then put under a microscope, and scrutinized to determine the stage of growth. It can also be used to identify a problem of anagen, systemic or telogen diseases. Telogen hairs have tiny bulbs growing from their roots that lack sheds. When you look at telogen effluvium, it is characterized by a higher proportion of hairs. Anagen hairs are covered with sheaths at their roots. Anagen effluvium is known to have a an abundance of broken hairs and an increase in hairs of the telogen phase.

Light microscopy - The physician uses a specific instrument that will examine all hairs which have been cut off at the base. This test is helpful because it allows you to discover any possible hair shaft issues.

Trichoscopy: This is a non-invasive method of looking at your hair and scalp. The test could be carried out with the help of a video dermoscope or handheld dermoscope. Most of the time, it permits a different diagnosis in the case of loss of hair.

Hair loss tests for other causes

Daily hair counts is usually done after the pull test results are negative. It is done by calculating the number of hairs that are lost. It is recommended to take note of the hair that was lost since the morning's first combing or after you wash for 14 days. Then, place it in a clean plastic bag. Keep track of the hair's strands. If the loss of hair exceeds 100 per day it's thought to be abnormal, except after shampooing when hair loss can be as high as 250 and still is considered normal.

For the majority of us when the idea to seek treatment natural treatments comes to mind we would like to conceal the fact that we have lost our hair. If you're still at this point Here are some suggestions to disguise your hair loss.

The Hair Loss Hideous

Head

You can conceal the loss of your hair by wearing an apron or hair piece such as a toupee, or hair wig. A hair wig is synthetic or natural hair that is created to look like the normal hairstyle. The hair is usually synthetic in the majority of cases, but sometimes it could be natural. This is why they differ widely in terms of cost and quality.

Another technique you can employ to cover up or conceal hair loss is "combing your hair" that is typically styling the hair that's been left over to cover the hair loss. However, this is an ineffective solution and only effective if the areas of balding are small. The comb-over loses its effectiveness when the loss of your hair is increasing.

Eyebrows

The loss of eyebrow hair isn't like loss of hair around the neck. A hormonal imbalance, chemotherapy, and other causes can result in the loss the eyebrow's hair. The best way to hide the loss of hair is by replacing your eyebrows by putting on artificial eyebrows. Another alternative is to use eyebrow embroidery. In this case, you make use of a knife to apply pigment to the eyebrows.

If you wish for the appearance to last You can choose the micropigmentation (permanent tattooing of makeup) option.

What is the cause of hair loss?

Every person loses between 50 and 100 hair strands every everyday, this is normal. If you're losing more than the above numbers of hair strands, it may be a serious issue. The loss of hair could be an indication of more serious medical conditions you aren't aware of. Therefore, it's essential to consult your doctor right away if you notice you're losing some hair. The treatment for losing hair is often different because the reasons for hair loss are different. The fact that the reasons are distinct has led to the creation of a lot of myths among those trying to explain the reason why they are losing hair. We will look at the truth behind these myths and look at the actual causes for hair loss, so that you can be able to find a solution in a more thorough manner.

Myths about Hair Loss

There are a myriad of myths about the loss of hair that ought be aware of to ensure you don't fall for a scam. The myths are:

* Diets can lead to hair loss

A balanced diet is suitable for general health. The absence of evidence-based studies has shown that certain food items result in hair loss. But, a severely restricted calorie diet or diets with low protein could cause temporary hair loss.

The loss of hair is a result of the mother's side

However, this isn't the case as, although the gene responsible for hair loss is linked to the x chromosome factors play an important role in the loss of hair. Research suggests that if someone has an unbald father and bald, he will likely eventually go through the same process.

* Wearing hats may strain the hair follicles. This can cause hair fall out

If you are a frequent wearer of a hat and you wear a hat often, there is no need to be concerned about your hair starting to fall out. The most important thing to do is that you wear an unclean hat since an unclean one could result in an infection of the scalp that can make it more difficult to lose hair.

* If you're experiencing baldness then you're old.

In contrast, teenagers and individuals in their 20s and 30s can be affected by the process of balding. However, the sooner it is noticed and the more severe it'll be.

* Exposed to sunlight causes hair loss.

Excessive exposure to the sun could cause skin issues, but it is not a cause for hair loss. Tannin beds are also not able to cause one to go bald.

* Men who are sexually active go bald at first

This isn't true because research has shown that men who are bald don't have more testosterone than those not bald.

The loss of hair every day is a sign that you're bald.

It is true that you lose hair every day if you suffer from male pattern hair loss. But, it's normal to lose up to 100 hairs a day because they usually regenerate.

The excessive washing of hair can to lead to loss of hair

Hair washing frequently doesn't necessarily cause loss of hair however, it is more likely to cause excessive manipulation that is done when hair is damp. We all know that hair becomes weak when it is wet therefore, if constantly wash your hair, it will need often detangle your hair, resulting in small loss of hair. The hair grows back quickly.

* Weave and weaves can cause hair loss

The majority of people believe that hair breathes and if it doesn't then it could lead to loss of hair. This is not true as hair doesn't need to breathe because the hair roots are the only thing living and receive oxygen from the blood in the scalp. Hairpieces such as wigs can cause harm if they're very tight.

* Female pattern hair loss can lead to irregular bleeding or irregular menstrual cycles

Hair loss is not a problem with endocrine function , menstrual problems. If you are experiencing hair loss and experience irregular bleeding, it could be an issue that is causing the issue, which could range from hormonal imbalances to diet to a lack of vitamins and minerals. It is recommended to have a blood test.

The use of a blow-dryer results in hair loss

There is no evidence that blow dryers cause hair to thin. But, excessive drying or high temperatures could cause breakable and brittle hair. Make sure you keep the dryer at a reasonable distance from your scalp, and dry it in an upward direction.

We've debunked the myths you might have heard about hair loss We'll now talk about the causes behind hair loss to help you distinguish fact from fiction:

Hair Loss Causes

What causes you to lose your hair more quickly than normal. This is why it is crucial to study the various reasons for hair loss to determine the best solutions for various causes of hair loss.

* Hair loss due to genetics

Genetic hair loss is known as androgenetic alopecia. It is among the most common causes of loss of hair. The gene is inherited from either the father's side or mom's side. It is more probable to be much more prominent when both your parents carry it.

For women, hairline could appear to be thinning around the bangs, and it could extend to the whole scalp. To determine if the reason behind the loss of hair is genetically based, a dermatologist typically observes the pattern of loss of hair. Other tests could include taking a scalp biopsy and a biopsy of the scalp to determine whether miniaturized follicules have replaced hair follicles. If you are suffering from inherited hair loss it is not always possible to cure hair loss because it's part of your genetic make-up However, you can reduce the process.

* Medical medical

Being afflicted by certain medical conditions can increase your risk of experiencing hair loss.

For instance, if suffer from thyroid issues then you could have suffered hair loss because the thyroid gland regulates hormone levels. Therefore when it's not functioning correctly it is possible to lose hair.

Ringworm infections, such as ringworm, can also cause hair loss.

Other skin issues, like certain forms of lupus could cause permanent loss of hair. Alopecia areata is one of the most common skin conditions. Alopecia areata can result in loss of hair since the condition is caused by the hair follicles get damaged by your immune system, leading to tiny round areas of loss of hair. Additionally, medications to treat medical conditions such as hypertension (beta-adrenergic blockers) as well as cancer (chemotherapy drugs) and arthritis (calcium channel blockers) and depression (antidepressants) are also recognized to cause hair loss. Birth medication for control and blood thinners can also cause temporary loss of hair. So, you must be aware if using any medication to treat these ailments.

Polycystic ovarian syndrome can also be an extremely commonly cited cause of loss of hair. More than five million women in the United States suffer from this condition. It can be diagnosed at 11 years old. It's usually due to hormonal imbalances where the ovaries create too many male hormones. Being afflicted with PCOS can lead to infertility. One of the most common signs of this disorder is when you begin to notice a growth in facial hair and irregular menstrual periods. Then, you may shed hair from your head but there may be hair growing on other areas of your body.

* Hair pulling disorder

This is typically a type of mental illness which makes people have an irresistible desire to pull their hair out. It could involve pulling hair out of hairline, the scalp or even other body parts. The continual pulling of hair may cause bald spots to appear on the hair.

* Physical or emotional shock

Certain people also notice hair loss over a period of time following an emotional or physical trauma. If something drastic happens to you and you begin to notice a loss of your hair, you should not be concerned, since the phase will go away. It is important to figure out ways to manage the loss of hair.

* Certain hairstyles

A lot of women have hairstyles that pull the hair too tight. So, having cornrows buns, and pigtails could cause hair loss due to traction.

Make sure your hair isn't pulled too tightly when making in a cornrow or weaving. Although these styles might seem attractive, they could cause a lot of damage if you experience hair loss as a result of certain actions.

* X-rays and injuries, as well as burns

This can lead to temporary loss of hair, and normal hair growth returns once the injury heals, unless you create scars, in which event your hair will never grow again.

* Cosmetic procedures

Too often washing your hair coloring, bleaching, dyeing and perms cause thinness of hair, making your hair dry and weak. The hair that you run through is often brittle and weak. curls, tight braiding , and rollers or curlers that are hot can cause damage and breakage to your hair, but they won't cause hair loss. Hair grows back normally when the issue is treated generally. However, hair loss or damage to the scalp hair loss can lead to permanent patches of hair loss.

* Hormones

Hormonal changes caused by menopausal issues, thyroid disorders childbirth, and pregnancy may result in permanent or temporary loss of hair.

* Risk factors

We've covered the causes of hair loss earlier however there are several factors that can increase your chances of experiencing hair loss.

They comprise:

* Stress

Weight loss is significant.

* Age

* Certain medical conditions , such as Lupus

* Family background of balding

What are the indications of a hair loss issues? It's not just about finding hair on your combs in the morning, is it? Let's look at these issues:

Affects and Signs Of Hair Loss

Loss of hair may occur in a variety of ways, according to the cause. It can occur slowly or suddenly , and it could be temporary or permanent. The symptoms and signs include:

* Scaling patches expanding over the scalp

These patches of scaling can be a sign of ringsworm. In these cases you may notice other signs as broken hair swelling, redness and even bleeding.

* Round or patchy spots

Some people have smooth bald spots that are that are the size of coins, and typically affects the scalp, but may affect beards, eyebrows, or even the hair. In certain cases the skin may become itchy or painful prior to the time that hair begins to fall out.

* Full-body hair loss

It is typically an outcome of illnesses and treatments. For example treatment with chemotherapy (for cancer) can cause hair loss throughout your body. Fortunately, hair typically recovers.

* Rapid loosening of hair

A physical or emotional trauma can cause hair to fall out. Hair strands may fall out when you wash your hair or combing it after gentle pulling. The loss of hair doesn't cause the appearance of bald patches, but rather general hair loss.

* Slowly thinning over the top of head

For females, forehead hair remains hairline, but the remaining portion of the hair shows an increase in size, whereas for men the hair begins receding at the forehead and forming an M-shaped line when they get older.

It is essential to know that losing hair isn't an all-purpose, one size that fits all. It can be seen in a variety of ways and we'll discuss them in the next section.

Chapter 3: Different types of Hair

Loss

Before deciding on any treatment method one of the primary steps that anyone suffering from alopecia should do is to determine the kind of hair loss the patient suffers from. In general, alopecia is characterized by excessive hair loss that causes an uneven or patchy loss of hair or balding on the scalp or other regions of the body, where hair growth is normally occurring.

But, as we discussed in the previous section of this book the loss of hair is caused by many diverse factors. To be able to determine the best treatment, it's the root of the problem that needs to be dealt with the utmost importance. It is important to identify precisely the kind of loss of hair that one suffers from so that you can be on the right path to the proper treatment.

The Most common types of hair loss

Androgenic Alopecia

Sometimes referred to in the context of male pattern baldness, or female pattern hair loss, androgenic Alopecia is a form of hair loss that is genetic causes. The most well-known kind of hair loss that happens for both genders androgenic alopecia is a condition that has genetic characteristics, which means that someone suffering from this disorder has acquired the tendency to lose hair through their ancestors.

Alopecia Areata

Alopecia areata can be described as a distinct kind of autoimmune disorder that occurs when the hair follicles get attacked by the body's self-defense system. The normal growth of hair is affected, which results in noticeable bald patches on the scalp. In some instances, on other body parts too.

Anagen Effluvium

The type of loss of hair is caused by the loss of hair due of the body's exposure to radiation, chemicals or toxins. The condition is usually experienced in the anagen stage period, which is the stage of growth in the lifecycle of hair. Anagen effluvium usually results in either a complete or partial loss of scalp hair as well as other body parts, such as eyebrows, eyelashes and various hairs on the body. Specific examples of the circumstances that could trigger anagen effluvium are certain types of cancer treatment, such as chemotherapy.

Telogen Effluvium

In this particular form of hair loss, hair follicles begin to move into the resting stage of the hair's lifespan which leads to the loss of hair. Telogen effluvium may be caused by illness, stress and other serious conditions that may cause strain on the body.

Trichotillomania

Trichotillomania is an impulse control disorder, which is sometimes called hair-pulling disorder. People with this disorder are prone to feeling an intense and uncontrollable desire to pull their hair out particularly when they're feeling stressed. It is common for this disorder to cause the loss of hair in the scalp as well as eyebrows and eyelashes.

There are many kinds of hair loss than those described within this section. Knowing more about these different kinds is an essential step to treatment. It is highly advised to seek with a medical professional to pinpoint the specific situation you're experiencing.

Chapter 4: Hair Care Home Remedies

The most effective way to combat loss of hair and encourage growth of hair is with natural solutions because they are secure and highly efficient. Explore your home because there are ways to get healthier, thicker and longer-lasting hair. These remedies at home include massaging your scalp and using the oils, herbs, and vegetables. They improve blood circulation, add nutrients into your hair and stimulate the sebaceous glands.

It is recommended to massage your hair with your fingertips (NOT FINGERNAILS) and OLIVE OIL. With vigor, but using a light pressure, massage the oil onto your scalp until the scalp is warm and begins to feel tingling. Massages stimulate sebaceous glands, and also stimulates the flow of blood towards your scalp. In the past, this will reduce and stop the loss of hair in the future.

One of the most effective methods to stop loss of hair, encouraging growth and keeping hair from graying is to make and applying homemade mustard seed or henna oil in your hair. (combine the two with healthy diet for hair health and you'll be getting close toward healthy hair!) Let's get started! ...

Take one cup of mustard oil and heat it in an oil skillet. Add four tablespoons of dried henna into the oil. You can also make use of henna powder, in the event that it is there is. As the oil boils, you'll notice bubbling that is active. Be cautious and take the pan off the flame immediately if you see bubbles that look like they're about to pop out from the pan. After that, lower the heat and place back on the high heat to keep it boiling, but give you to control the process.

If the oil ceases to bubble this means that all water-based moisture has been removed from the mix (the process usually takes between 30 and 40 minutes).

Remove the heat from the stove and allow to cool at least a few minutes.

After the oil has cooled slightly, but it is warm and viscusy, place a towel to filter the oil onto a dry, clean glass jar that is large enough to accommodate all the ingredients of your fry pan. Be sure to use the jar with lid. Pour the oil on the cloth, and allow it to run down into the container.

After you are done when you are done, let the jar of oil cool to ambient temperature. Then, take off the cloth , then put the lid back on. Then store at the room temperature.

Once you are prepared to make use of the oil just warm it by placing an amount of it into a microwave-safe dish. Then cook the dish at medium setting until it's warm (start with about 10 seconds of heating and then reheat it in case that's not sufficient time for warming the oil). If you'd rather, instead of using the microwave, you can immerse the jar into hot water (be cautious not to allow water in the jar since it can get in the oil). You can test your oil's temperature using your finger or by placing a small drop of oil on your wrist. If it's a pleasant temperature, rub the oil into your locks and the scalp.

Repeat this process at least every two to three days to get the best results.

Another option is cut some onion slices and apply them to your scalp until the hairy patches change color. Make use of honey and apply this to relax and awaken your scalp. Repeat this every throughout the day, particularly at evening and in the morning. (You might need to research this more thoroughly, since honey is known to be very sticky. Perhaps somebody could give tips on how you can make use of this product with less clutter. Please let me know if you have it!)

Margosa is a great herb to prevent hair loss, encourage hair growth, improve color , and eliminate parasites. Find a tablespoon of leaves and mix them with one cup of water inside a tiny vessel with lid. For 3 to five minutes, allow the mixture to simmer. The lid should be covered as it simmers. The liquid left over should be separated (removing any leaves) into the cup or bowl. Mix in honey to enhance the flavor, and then drink the mixture. This treatment can be used daily to remove hair loss.

Take the black pepper seeds along with lime, and then grind them into an emulsion. Apply the paste to areas of your scalp that hair loss is occurring. Expect your scalp to become slightly irritated, but this will boost the flow of blood to it, specifically the areas with hair loss or patches of baldness. If your blood flow increases it will increase the amount of nutrients transferred to the hair follicles, which will increase the growth of your hair. Do this 2 times a every day for the duration of one month.

Use these simple home remedies now to see your hair growing and growing healthier.

Chapter 5: The Hair Replacement and Wigs

It is another option to treat hair loss issues. Hair replacements that don't need surgery are a great option if the goal is to restore the look of longer hair without having to go under the surgical knife. It's not a crime to do it and the stigma associated with it has diminished significantly in recent years as many people are wearing hair wigs.

Wigs aren't only for those who are not bald or have spots of baldness. Celebrities with hair that is full are wearing wigs to make a fashion appearance. Many people are looking to alter their appearance without cutting their hair. Coloring your hair and styling and wearing wigs is among the options to achieve this.

Hairpieces can be purchased comprised of human hair, and they are easy to locate these on the internet. But, if you're not sure of what you should look for prior to making a purchase Here are a few tips on how to choose the perfect hair replacement that is right for you:

BASE MATERIALS

There are three types of base materials utilized by a variety of manufacturers to create their hair replacement products. There are mesh bases, polymer bases or even a mix of both.

Wigs made of polymer are more durable and easy to fix, and cheaper. Polymer meshes consist from either silicone or polyurethane and are intended to mimic the appearance of the hair. However, wigs made from polymer could be uncomfortable to wear as they can get hot.

A hair replacement item with a mesh fabric base is more natural looking and can be virtually unnoticeable. Mesh-fabric wigs are easier to put on as they're lightweight and cool.

Mesh fabric can be constructed of polyester or nylon and this is the reason hairline that is fine can be made out of this material. The downside to these wigsis that they cost more, are less durable, require regular replacement, and may react with body chemical reactions in a negative way. Other wigs make use of a mixture of mesh and polymer. They will differ in terms of size as well as comfort, appearance and cost. Therefore, you should locate a base for your hairpiece that is comfortable for you.

The most important thing to consider before buying Make sure to look for possibility of problems

using the hairpiece. If the offer is too appealing in reality, it most likely is. If you are able to test it to observe how your body react to the substance that is the item, try it.

HAIR

We all know that there are hairpieces that are made of human hair. Certain companies will even provide you hair pieces that are of such high-end quality that it will be exactly like your hair! Then it's not only the color that matches as well, the curl, wave and the texture the hair's texture will also match also. Some even be able to match the volume that your hair has. However, this type of hairpiece is bound to be costly.

Today, there are more affordable hairpiecesthat are available and although they may contain human hair inside but it's not the complete hairpiece. Certain hairpieces will contain a mix of animal and human hair, while others contain artificial and human hair.

Hairpieces with the highest price are created in Europe and come in a range of densities, colors, styles, and textures (straight curly, straight or curly or). The cheapest hairpieces are manufactured in Asia as they tend to be black and straight.

Hairpieces can be secured with clips or adhesives. If you decide to make use of an adhesive, you should be aware that it can increase the loss of hair especially in the area that the bond is applied. Clips aren't as destructive, however they're not the safest method of attaching your hairpiece.

There are methods for your hairpieces to be semi-permanent. But, they need to be positioned to your head by stylists or hair technicians and should be changed each six-week period. Hair is attached with different liquid adhesives. Some have temporary adhesives and for hairpieces with these, the double-sided tape could be employed.

Chapter 6: Home Remedies

Lemon

Lemon is widely used for the treatment of various kinds of hair-related issues, including the cradle cap condition, hair loss and dry hair among other issues. Follow these steps to utilize lemon to treat hair loss:

Add 1 tablespoon of juice from a lemon into around 2 teaspoons olive oil.

Apply the mixture to your hair

After a while then rinse the area with mild shampoo. It is possible to repeat this three times per week for positive results.

Egg Yolk

Mix egg yolk and honey , then apply the mixture to the patches of hair that are bald. Allow it to sit for around 30 minutes, then wash it off. This will strengthen your hair.

Egg yolks can also be applied plainly to your scalp. You can do this by beating an egg yolk inside a bowl until the texture is silky and smooth. Rub it onto your scalp and let it dry at least 30 mins. Rinse and wash your hair with cool water.

Honey

Honey is a great solution for treating different hair related issues such as loss of hair, baldness, or dry hair. Simply make a mixture of 2 tablespoons honey, 2 tablespoons of olive oil warm and 1 teaspoon of powdered cinnamon. Allow it to sit for 20 minutes and then rinse your hair using fresh water.

Bananas

Bananas are not just great for treating hair loss, but are also beneficial for skin. Bananas are also a remedy for other hair-related problems such as dry hair split endsand dandruff and other issues. This recipe is simple to make and makes healthy and nutritious snack. All you have to do is prepare the shake using yogurt and honey, as well as bananas along with skimmed or skimmed milk. Now you can enjoy your drink!

It is also possible to create a hair mask using avocado as well as banana. Mash 2 tablespoons of honey, two bananas, 3 tablespoons olive oil, 3 tablespoons of buttermilk, and a mashed avocado. Mix all the ingredients well and apply the mix to your hair strands as well as your scalp. Allow it to sit for around 20 minutes before washing with warm water.

Baking soda

For treatment for hair loss Take 3 cups of hot water , and then add two tablespoons of baking soda. Mix until baking soda disintegrates completely. Apply it like normal shampoo, by pouring it over your hair and massage it lightly.

You can also create a mask lemon juice, baking soda as well as baking soda. Mix this into a glass with shampoo that is filled to about 1/4 in the size of the container. Shake the mixture well and then use it like a regular shampoo. For best results, apply this method only one time within four weeks.

Coconut Milk

Coconut milk is rich in essential fats as well as protein which encourage hair growth and stop loss of hair. If you apply it on your hair it may deliver immediate results. Follow the steps below:

- Make coconut oil fresh by greasing a coconut, later adding it into an empty pan of water.

Let it simmer for around 5 minutes before straining it.

Allow it to cool and then apply the milk to your scalp and then in your hair. Let it sit for 20 minutes and then proceed to wash your hair.

You can increase the efficacy for the remedy by mixing powdered fenugreek and pepper in coconut milk prior to using it.

Black Pepper

Black pepper is a powerful treatment for hair loss and baldness. loss. Preparing treatment:

Making a smooth paste crushing/grinding the black pepper with the lime seeds until a fine paste has made.

The paste should be applied directly on your scalp and apply it out evenly.

Leave it on for a few minutes, then wash it off. If it begins to hurt then stop using the treatment right away.

Red Gram as well as Pigeon Pea

Red gram can be used to reduce hair loss. It can be made more effective by adding pigeonpea. For preparing a remedy grind the pigeon pea along with red gram to create an extremely thin paste. Apply the paste to areas that are bald to promote hair growth and prevent loss of hair.

To make sure that you do not lose your hair again It is essential to understand how to take take care of the hair. The next chapter will provide ways to take proper care of your hair to avoid losing hair.

Chapter 7: Sweet Themed Shampoos

There is no way to resist the taste of strawberries and chocolate gateaux, however people don't want the calories that accompany the dessert. You can however make an exquisite range of homemade shampoos with a theme that make your saliva flow and your scales breathe in relief.

Hair Shampoo with Hot Chocolate (best to use only on hair with black or brown color)

1/4 cup of water distilled

1 cup of castile soap that is unscented.

One tablespoon chocolate oil essential

1/2 tablespoon cocoa powder

1 empty, clean bottle

Directions

Mix all the ingredients together and put them in the clean bottle and shake until the ingredients are well blended. Before use, shake thoroughly.

Chocolate Mint (best to use only on black or brown hair)

1/4 cup of water distilled

1 cup of castile soap that is unscented.

One tablespoon chocolate oil essential

1 tablespoon of essential peppermint oils

1 empty, clean bottle

Directions

Mix all the ingredients together and place them into the clean bottle and shake until the ingredients are well mixed. Before use, shake thoroughly.

Ginger Peach Shampoo

1/4 cup of water distilled

1 cup of castile soap that is unscented.

1 tablespoon of essential oils from ginger

1 tablespoon of essential oils of the peach

1 empty, clean bottle

Directions

Mix all the ingredients together and put them in the bottle that is clean and empty and shake until the ingredients are well combined. Before use, shake thoroughly.

A luxurious salted caramel shampoo

1/4 cup of water distilled

1 cup of castile soap that is unscented.

One tablespoon caramel oil essential

1/2 teaspoon of salt

1 empty, clean bottle

Directions

Mix all the ingredients together and put them in the clean bottle and shake until the ingredients are well mixed. Before use, shake thoroughly.

Amazing Strawberry Shake Shampoo

1/4 cup of water distilled

1 cup of castile soap that is unscented.

One tablespoon shampoo oil essentials

1 cup milk

1 empty bottle that is clean and clean.

Directions

Gather all the ingredients and put them in the bottle that is clean and empty and shake until the ingredients are well blended. Before use, shake thoroughly.

Crazy Cotton Candy Shampoo

1/4 cup of water distilled

1 cup of castile soap that is unscented.

1 tablespoon of essential oils from cotton candy

1 tablespoon essential sweet almond oils

1 empty, clean bottle

Directions

Gather all the ingredients and put them in the clean bottle and shake until the ingredients are well blended. Before use, shake thoroughly.

Fantastic Orange as well as Vanilla shampoo

1/4 cup of water distilled

1 cup of castile soap that is unscented.

1 tablespoon of essential orange oils

1 tablespoon French vanilla essential oils

1 empty, clean bottle

Directions

Mix all the ingredients together and put them into the clean bottle and shake until the ingredients are well blended. Prior to use, shake the bottle thoroughly.

Chapter 8: Ayurvedic Cures

Ayurvedic treatments aren't as fast when compared with alopathic treatments, however they are less expensive and have a lasting effect. There are many remedies and herbs found that are part of ayurveda to reverse the loss of hair. A few of these are listed as follows..

1). Onion - Rich in antibacterial as well as antifungal qualities, using onion to treat hair loss keep hair loss at bay. Here are 10 incredible ways to benefit your hair from onions:

They're very effective in the nourishment of hair follicles and replenish the nutrients that have been lost to your scalp.

They're rich in Sulphur that is thought to prevent breakage and reduce thinning.

They possess potent antibacterial properties and can fight off scalp infections. This helps to slow the loss of hair because scalp infections can cause the loss of hair to a large extent.

They are powerful antioxidants naturally found in nature This is the reason they are able to in reversing the effects of premature graying.

This vegetable gives a natural shine and health to your hair that can last for a long time if it is used frequently.

Researchers have discovered that they are able to protect the head and neck from cancers of the head and neck.

They also make your hair unsuitable for lice.

Make your hair look more full by adding onion juice to style your hair.

They can also be used in the fight against dandruff because of their powerful anti-bacterial properties.

They increase blood circulation, which can help to increase hair growth.

Learn to Make Onion Juice At-Home

Peel the onions, then cut them into four parts.

Blend them with a juicer or grinder

Make sure to add a bit of water, then strain the juice with the cotton cloth.

This will make sure that no onion pieces remain in your hair when you are using the juice.

Learn how to use onion Juice to increase hair growth

Give your scalp a thorough treatment with onion juice

Utilizing your fingers gentle massage the scalp your scalp with circular motions

Allow it to rest for approximately. 1 hour.

Rinse it out by using a mild, mild shampoo with pleasant scent to eliminate the strong onion scent. Pantene Pro-V Silky Smooth care shampoo and conditioner clean your hair without causing irritation and provide nourishment.

Try this regularly to see the results. You could try it every week for two months and see a visible changes.

You could also include onion's benefits and other ingredients to make better, more shiny hair!

4 homemade onion juice hair Packs for Healthier, Stronger Hair

1 Honey and Onion Juice Hair Growth Pack Hair Growth

Take quarter cup onion juice

Combine a teaspoon of honey into this juice

Apply this mix to your hair's scalp and hair roots.

Rinse it off after 30 mins with mild shampoo

2 Olive Oil and Onion Juice Hair Massage to promote hair growth

Olive oil is an excellent oil to use for massages on your hair because it penetrates the scalp and provides it with nourishment. It also contains anti-dandruff characteristics which is an added benefit!

3 tablespoons of onion juice.

Include 1 and half tablespoons olive oil into it.

Massage this mixture on your scalp using circular motions

Rinse it off with a gentle shampoo after two hours.

Keep doing this on a regular basis to build healthier, smoother hair!

#3 Onion and Curry Leaves Hair Mask

Curry leaves are known for its numerous benefits to hair. It aids in strengthening hair, reduces greying and promotes healthy hair.

Mix fresh curry leaves into a paste

2. Add two tablespoons of juice from onions to this curry paste.

Use this hair pack to your scalp

Clean it off using mild shampoo after about an hour.

#4 Onion and Yogurt Hair Pack to Strengthen Hair

Yogurt is a great food to fight hair fall and, when mixed to onion juice, aids in the process of growing hair.

Mix 2 tablespoons yogurt and the juice of an onion in the bowl of.

Use this mask to your scalp

Rinse this mix off using gentle shampoo after about an hour.

Tips to remember when using Onion Juice:

Make sure to filter the juice to keep out the flaky onion particles that are inside your hair. Eliminating these flaky bits from your hair will be an unpleasant job. It is better to separate the juice using the help of a muslin cloth prior to applying it to the scalp.

Use mild shampoos to remove onion juice out of your hair.

You can add garlic or apple cider vinegar for the added benefits from these ingredients.

If you aren't able to stand the strong smell it is possible to add a few drops one of your preferred essential oils to the juice.

Always conduct a patch test prior to using onion juice

2). Aloe Vera2. Aloe Vera Aloe vera is the best hair you could ever get. It is a huge source of amino acids and proteolytic enzymes that effectively to improve the health of your scalp and increase hair growth. To help make the process of growing hair much easier I've compiled fifteen different ways to utilize aloe vera to increase hair growth. Before we get started, let's take a examine how aloe vera helps hair.

A lot of people inquire "is aloe vera beneficial for hair?" And "what does aloe vera do to the hair?" The answer to the first question is "Yes!" Aloe vera is wonderful for hair! It may sound like I'm exaggerating, however, aloe vera is actually among the top amazing and effective ingredients you can apply to your hair. Are you skeptical? It's not necessary to. However, you shouldn't be able to argue with the facts...

As I've mentioned previously the aloe vera plant contains proteolytic enzymes that help heal and repair damaged hair's cells. This improves the health of your hair follicles and in turn promotes healthy hair growth and speed.

Not only can the proteolytic enzyme aid in healing the scalp however, it can also help revive dormant hair follicles by encouraging hair growth.

It also aids in reducing hair loss and prevents hair loss, ensuring your hair stays thick and full.

It contains anti-inflammatory properties that will soothe your scalp of irritation and irritation.

The antiviral as well as antifungal properties aid in combat flaking and dandruff.

Aloe vera's abundance of vitamins, protein, and minerals aid in nourishing your hair's follicles.

The aloe vera aids in conditioning your hair, securing the nutrients and hydration.

Once you've answered your questions Let's take a look at the various ways to use the aloe-vera plant in your hair-care routine.

1. Castor Oil And Aloe Vera to promote hair growth

You'll Need

1 cup Fresh Aloe Vera Gel

2 Tbsp Castor Oil

2 Tbsp Fenugreek Powder

Shower Cap

Towel

A bowl is used to mix the ingredients until you've got an even and smooth paste.

Apply the mixture on your hair and scalp. Make sure you're focused on your hair's roots and tips.

When your hair is completely coated in the mix Cover the hair by a cap for showers.

You can sleep with the mix in the bed. You could put a towel over the cap of your shower to provide warmth and to prevent the cap from moving.

The next day, wash the mix off using cold soap and water. Follow with conditioner.

How often?

2 or 3 times per each week.

What is the reason? This How It Works

Castor oil is a fantastic treatment for hair growth. It helps increase hair growth and increasing volume. The oil, along with aloe-vera can help stimulate hair growth and reduces the fall of hair. The aloe vera treatment can to stimulate growth of hair from hair follicles that are dormant on your scalp. It can also help maintain and nourish hair strands, which can prevent breaks and splitting of ends.

2).Honey and Aloe Vera To Increase Hair Growth

You'll Have

5 tbsp Aloe Vera Gel

3 Tbsp Coconut Oil

2 Tbsp Honey

Shower Cap

Prep Time

5 minutes

Processing Time

25 minutes

Process

A bowl is the best place to mix all the ingredients until you have an even mix.

Begin by massaging this mix onto your scalp. Then apply it to the ends of your hair. Concentrate on the tips because they are the areas that are most damaged on your head.

When all your hair has been covered with the mix, put a cap over your shower and leave it on for approximately 25 minutes.

Shampoo your hair using cold shampoo and water. Follow with conditioner.

How often?

Every week, once.

The Reasons This Why It Works

Honey and coconut oil are an excellent combination for conditioning, which aids in sealing moisture into the hair shafts. This mask can aid in maintaining your hair, which means you won't require haircuts as often, and let you maintain the length of your hair.

3. Egg and Aloe Vera for Hair Growth

You'll Be In Need

4 tbsp Fresh Aloe Vera Gel

3 Tbsp Olive Oil

1 Egg Yolk

Shower Cap

Prep Time

5 minutes

Processing time

25 minutes

Process

Mix in a bowl the ingredients until you have an even, smooth paste.

Apply the mixture on your hair and scalp. Be sure to focus on your tips and roots.

When your hair is completely coated with the mixture then cover the hair using a cap for showers.

The mixture should be left on for 20 to 25 minutes.

Rinse the mixture using cold soap and water. It is not recommended to make use of warm water as it can cook the egg in the mixture.

Finish by applying conditioner.

How often?

Each week, you will be able to do it.

What is the reason? This Why It Works

The egg's yolk is full of fats making it a potent conditioning ingredient. When combined together with aloe and olive oils it aids in nourishing your hair and increase the speed that your hair is growing.

4. Onion And Aloe Vera For Hair Growth

You'll need

1 Cup Onion Juice

1 Tbsp Aloe Vera Gel

Prep Time

10 minutes

Processing Time

1 hour

Process

Take around 3-4 onions, and then blend into an emulsified form in a blender. Utilize a cheesecloth for removing the juice.

In the juice include the gel of aloe vera, and mix it well.

Massage the mixture onto your scalp and move on your hair, ensuring that it is completely soaked in the liquid.

Let it sit for approximately an hour, and then proceed to wash your hair.

Cleanse your hair using mild shampoo, and then end with conditioner.

How often?

Each week, you will be able to do it.

What is the reason for this work?

It is among the most intense treatments for hair growth. It can help stop hair loss and stimulates hair growth. Onion juice is a great hair growth ingredient , stimulating your scalp and dormant follicles thereon. A regular use of this mask will result in impressive length and the thickness.

3).Bhringraj for hair loss - Bhringraj, or Eclipta Alba, is a well-known herb that is renowned for its health advantages. Bhringraj offers so many benefits for hair that in products for hair care also this herb is utilized extensively. Bhringraj oil as well as bhringraj powder are utilized for hair care particularly when hair loss is observed. This amazing herb is extensively utilized for Ayurevdic treatments. It is loaded with vital minerals and vitamins that help to boost hair growth and improve blood circulation.

What is the reason Bhringraj is good for Hair?

Bhringraj is extremely beneficial for the dull and dry hair since it deeply nourishes the hair.

It also improves blood flow on the scalp, which provides relief from the loss of hair and also stimulates the scalp to encourage the growth of new hair.

It can also help with the fight against dandruff, and controlling lice-related parasites.

With the aid of bhrinraj hair care products, you can have silky and shiny hair.

This medication stops hair loss and loss of hair very rapidly when used frequently.

It is also believed that bhringraj helps with migraine and headache.

Additionally, this herb helps to prevent premature hair loss and graying.

Bhringraj (Eclipta Alba) for hair fall and loss of hair

Below are the main remedies that include bhringraj, as well as other natural remedies to combat your hair loss and loss issues.

1. Bhringraj Oil Treatment

Oiling your hair is vital to maintain the well-being that your hair enjoys. Oiling with Bhringraj oil offers nourishment as well as deeply conditions your hair and its roots. It is a source of anti-oxidants and vitamins that are contained in the oil in the hair. To avoid significant loss of hair and early graying, use bhringraj oil. This helps to reduce dryness and loss of hair. Oils such as almond oil and olive oil are beneficial in removing hair loss and ill health.

You can make Bhringraj oil from coconut oil. Or purchase the oil in the shops.

How do you create Bhringraj oils for hair?

Drink half a cup of Bhringraj leaves.

In a pan, heat the oil with 1 cup coconut oil.

Once the oil is warm then add the leaves to the oil.

Let it boil. This will help the leaves of bhringraj to release their extracts to the coconut oil.

Cook for another 4-5 minutes and then reduce the heat.

Allow the oil to cool. Mash the leaves using fingers, and then strain the oil.

This oil is strained and is Bhringraj coconut oil.

What is the best way to use this oil?

In the evening, divide the hair in two sections.

Massage the oil on the scalp for several minutes.

Then follow it to the tips and ends.

Put on a shower cap and tie your hair into a top knot

Let it rest for a night and rinse it off using shampoo.

Make sure to apply an oil conditioner afterward.

Hair loss can be prevented by using this fantastic hair pack. It is made up of yoghurt and black pepper and bhringraj leaf. We know that Bhringraj can be helpful in stopping the recurrence of hair loss and damage to hair. Yoghurt has essential fat acids as well as vitamins such vitamin C and vitamin A. Black pepper causes black hair color and provides relief from the itching and dandruff. It makes hair stronger and shiny.

How do you create it?

Make 1 cup of fresh yogurt and put it in the bowl.

Mix it thoroughly so that there aren't any lumps present.

Also, take 20-30 leaves of bhringraj and clean them.

Then, grind them in the grinder, adding a little water. This will create a dense paste.

Place it into the same bowl.

Then add a half teaspoon of black pepper crushed in this bag.

Mix everything thoroughly and it's now ready for use.

Comb your hair in a proper manner and let them untangle.

Use a hair brush to apply this hair pack to the scalp and roots evenly.

Follow your hair's guidelines and the ends.

Do it for 25 minutes.

Clean it using a shampoo or conditioner.

3. Bhringraj along with Yoghurt Mask

Use 1/2 cup of bhringraj leaves and crush them in the grinder with a bit of water.

Add 1 cup of yoghurt or curd in the mix.

Mix it all up and then apply the mask on the scalp and hair

Rinse your hair every 2 hours.

Yoghurt creates new hair and helps reduce the hair loss.

4. Eggs, Lemon, and Bhringraj pack

Bhringraj along with Lemon are great for treating the loss of hair caused by the scalp being itchy and dandruffy.

Make 1/4 cup of Bhringraj paste and mix it in a bowl.

2. Add 2 teaspoons of juice from a lemon.

Add 1 egg, and beat the mixture to combine everything.

Apply this mask to your head and hair. Use for two hours.

Cleanse using cold water, and a mild soap afterwards.

Try this twice in the course of a week to prevent hair loss and fall in hair for both genders.

5. Bhringraj Fenugreek, Bhringraj, and Curd Mask

Incubate a quarter cup of fenugreek in the water in a bowl at midnight.

The next day, take the Fenugreek seeds, along with 1 cup of bhringraj powder or leaves.

Mix this up with water. It will form a paste.

In the paste, add a teaspoons of yoghurt.

Mix and apply to the scalp and hair.

Rinse hair after two hours.

Try it every week

.

6. Hibiscus flower and Bhringraj for hair growth

Use bhringraj leaves about 1/4 cup, and hibiscus flowers between 10-12.

Place them in the grinder and then, using water, grind them.

Incorporate some curd into this paste.

Make hair mask and leave for at least 1-2 hours.

After that, wash it off with simple water.

7. Curry Leaves and Bhringraj

Use 1/2 cup curry leaves, and 1/2 cup of bhringraj leaf or powder if bhringraj leaves are not readily available.

Mix them until you have the consistency of a paste.

Apply the paste to your scalp for one hour.

Rinse the hair using tepid water.

8. Onion Juice Coconut oil, and Bhringraj Oil

Take 2-3 teaspoons of coconut oil and 14 Cup of juice from onions.

In this, add 4-5 teaspoons of Bhringraj oil.

Mix the oil and massage it on your scalp.

Maintain this for at most 2 hours, then rinse using mild soap.

If the onion scent persists, then you can use lemon juice to give your hair a final wash.

9. Amla and Bhringraj

Take 3 teaspoons of amla powder and bhringraj powder per.

Mix them together using coconut water or even some water.

Apply the lotion and massage the scalp.

Rinse the hair using regular water.

Repeat the process twice a week to see results with hair loss and treating bald patches caused by Alopecia.

4). Garlic is a hair loss remedy.

Who doesn't like the scent of garlic that has been freshly cooked? Even if you don'tlike it, you must know that the ingredient can be used for more than being a garnish. For instance you can use it to increase the growth of hair. In an age that consumers are spending more and more money on treatments at salons as well as extensions naturally occurring ingredient has been deemed to be a hugely under-appreciated hair growth aid. Garlic's role as a hair treatment ingredient is able to not just boost hair growth but also to stimulate growth of hair. Here's how the root vegetable works it:

Garlic's benefits for hair Growth

Garlic is rich in of minerals, including zinc, calcium and sulfur. These are necessary for hair growth.

It's antimicrobial and can help fight off bacteria and germs which can cause harm to the scalp and impede hair growth.

The selenium-rich garlic can help increase blood flow to ensure optimal nutrition

It aids in cleansing the hair folliclesand strengthen them, and stop the hair from falling out.

It aids in calming irritated scalp and treat issues like dandruff

Raw garlic is incredibly loaded with Vitamin C that is excellent for your health and the condition and hair. It increases collagen production, which assists in the growth of hair.

Chapter 9: General Hair well-being and Stimulation

Laser Comb

Similar to other treatments to grow hair using so-called laser combs seems to function by stimulating blood flow to hair follicles. The process is called photo-biostimulation, which subjects the hair follicles to laser energy. The results of photo-biostimulation have shown that it can increase the amount of hair in the area of treatment in the course of time. The procedure is based on the use of the kind of comb which radiates the scalp with low-level laser light for a period of 10 to 15 minutes, a couple of times each week. It's not said to be a long-lasting or effective treatment for severe hair loss, however it has been shown to yield results, and works best when combined with other methods that have been proven to work.

Scalp Massage

Massaging the scalp increases the flow of blood into the hair follicles. The improved circulation of blood has been proved to be efficient in increasing the growth of hair and improving health. In fact many of the techniques which have been previously examined are believed to be beneficial by increasing blood circulation. The most successful results are when massage is utilized alongside other methods including the use of essential oils.

Personal Review

When you apply shampoo oils, hair oil, or other type of treatment applied to your hair's texture, instructions generally follow similar - massage your scalp. A boost in blood circulation allows for greater absorption of the product through the skin. If washing my hair using the products listed in the book, I make sure to massage my scalp. Making small circles using my fingers against my scalp, I usually begin either by rubbing my sideburns, moving up and around over the ears towards the back, and then upor towards my hairline in front. Self-massaging is also something I find very relaxing.

Propecia (Finasteride)

Finasteride is an antidepressant which was initially developed to reduce prostate glands that were enlarged. Strangely enough, there's evidence that suggests that an increased prostate size is due to hormonal imbalances such as androgens. These can also be linked to hair loss that is premature. Researchers found that Finasteride was able to assist in grow hair which is why it was developed further as an effective treatment for hair loss. It is believed to be effective due to its ability to block testosterone's conversion to DHT which is believed to be harmful for hair development. Finasteride treatment, when it is effective is a daily pill that can be used for an indefinite period of time. In the absence of development of new hair It may be able to aid in maintaining your hair that you currently have. Due to the variety of adverse effects, Finasteride is usually only available on prescription and should only be utilized under the guidance of a doctor.

Personal Review

This is a well-known option for reducing hair loss, but there is a significant adverse effect that every user or people who are considering it must be aware of. Consuming Propecia could cause Erectile dysfunction. There have been numerous studies conducted on Propecia since its introduction on the market and the most commonly reported adverse result being Erectile dysfunction. While this only affects 1 percent of male users, being aware of the possibility that this pill may cause harm to my sexual health and likely in the future the long-term, it was enough to turn me off using Propecia before I even consumed my first bottle. I would recommend taking caution when using this medication, and when considering the various alternatives offered, I'd suggest keeping clear of the pill.

Saw Palmetto Extract

Saw Palmetto Extract is derived from the fruits of Serenoa Repens, also known as the Saw Palmetto plant - which is a tiny palm indigenous in the Southeastern United States. The extract of Saw Palmetto block the testosterone-converting enzyme, which converts into DHT that is responsible for the loss of hair. The treatment is administered orally and , despite only a small amount of research to demonstrate its efficacy, it is still a common choice for treating hair loss. Also, be aware that it causes blood thinning and might necessitate the oversight of a doctor.

Personal Review

I used this supplement in my first times of concern about hair loss. Many men use Saw Palmetto in an effort to decrease prostate size. prostates, however, in my early 20s this was not a concern for me. I did experience small side effects, such as nausea and constipation that was irritable. The reviews suggest that this could be common when taking the supplement with a full stomach. However, even though I was taking one capsule every morning following breakfast, the typical side effects were evident. After a few months I was unable to see any improvement in my hair, so I decided to stop, however there are many people who have glowing reviews and good outcomes.

Shower Filter

Shower filters serve to remove chemicals and other contaminates from the water while bathing. A particular chemical, chlorine can cause skin to dry out and become unhealthy. Although dry skin isn't the cause of loss of hair but it could hinder the growth of healthy hair, and can hinder the efficacy of other treatments for hair loss.

Chapter 10: Natural Herbal Recipes For Healthy and Nourished Hair, As Well As Scalp

Hair is a reflection of the overall condition of the body. Hair that is healthy should extend by about 30% before it is broken. The body that is healthy an image that a scalp healthy as well as flowing hair. Herbs can aid in helping all hair types stay looking and feeling healthy. There are numerous natural herbs that can be used to treat hair, and they have been used in many nations for centuries today.

Here are a few of the most frequently used herbal ingredients that you can apply to your hair:

Aloe Vera Birch Arnica, Catmint Burdock, Horsetail, Chamomile, Marigold, Licorice, Nettles, Rosemary, Parsley, Southernwood, Sage, Chamomile, Stinging nettle, and Mulberries. Soy is equally important to stop loss of hair.

Certain herbal rinses can be used to treat scalp problems like dandruff, itching and flaky scalp. They can also help with oily scalp, and stunted growth. Herbs may help improve circulation to the scalp and speed up hair growth by stimulating of hair follicles.

A shampoo rinse is a affordable method to treat and strengthen your both hair and scalp.

Herbal Hair Rinses:

For hair loss and thinness: Burdock, Bhringraj, Amla, Fenugreek, Hops, Horsetail, Lavender, Nettle Red clover Rosemary, Sage, Shikakai, Thyme, Tulsi, Watercress, Yashtimadhu

To enhance the luster: Aloe vera, Basil, Aritha, Dandelion, Horsetail, Nettle, Parsley, Rosemary, Seaweed, Shikakai

To treat dry scalp and hair: Calendula Comfrey, Flaxseed (linseed), Ginger root, Lavender, Parsley, Sage

For scalps and hair with oily hair: Horsetail, Lavender, Lemon balm, Lemongrass Nettle

Peppermint, Rosemary, Thyme Watercress, Yarrow

For blond highlights: Chamomile, Mullein, Rhubarb root

For highlights in red: Hibiscus, Red clover and rose hips.

For dark highlights: Black tea, Coffee, Black walnut, Cloves, Comfrey, Rosemary, Sage

Hair rinse recipe using Burdock root to prevent loss of hair and encourage hair growth

Ingredients:

One teaspoon Burdock root

200ml of water

Directions

Boil the water along with the burdock root in a saucepan for 10 minutes. After that, let it sit with a cover on for an additional 20 minutes. Then strain the Burdock roots using the help of a strainer. Make use of the liquid as an end-of-day rinse for washed hair, or as a toner for the skin.

Pour the liquid into the spray bottle and then spray your scalp.

In the making of other natural hair shampoos, it is easy. Making the Nettle as well as the Rosemary rinse, it is the same as other infusions. You can add a tablespoon of herb in 300-500ml of boiling water. Then, under the cover, you can brew it for 10 to 15 minutes. Then strain the herb using an strainer and allow the water to cool. Apply it as a last rinse for freshly washed and conditioned hair.

Drinking lots of herbal teas, water as well as unsweetened juices of fruit can also help improve the health of your hair. Horsetail tea or Nettle tea are the best teas for hair growth. Consume it daily for three months. Once the time has passed, take a break for one month.

Collagen which is so crucial for a beautiful hair is discovered in Silica. Zine can help increase thyroid function and reduce the possibility of hair loss that is caused by an the thyroid gland being underactive. This Butterfly Pea herb was known as a key ingredient in Thai herbal medicines that can treat gray and hair loss. hair. Amla can be beneficial in restoring hair's natural acidity like the balance of alkaline. Shikakai as well as Reetha are beneficial and efficient in ensuring that hair is healthier.

Massage your scalp using warm almond oil or olive oil. Mix half a cup of water and two egg yolks and mix well. Make use of the mixture to massage on your hair and scalp for between five and 10 minutes. Apply it to your hair for a few minutes before you rinse it off with water that is lukewarm. Rinse with an apple cider vinegar as well as water that is clean. If you suffer from extremely dry hair, make elderflower brews parsley, sage, or. The frizzy hair will be restored to the moisture it has lost. If you're suffering from oily or greasy hair you can wash it using lemon balm mint, lavender, or rosemary. It is possible to combine lavender oil with coconut oil, and then boil it. When it cools, you can apply the oil to your scalp throughout the night, and then wash it using a natural shampoo the next morning.

Chapter 11: How to Avoid the Risks

to reduce hair loss

Don't style or style hair that is wet. If your hair is damp be careful not to style or brush the hair for as long as you can. Hair is weakest when it's wet. When hair that is wet is styled or brushed, it can result in maximum hair loss, even if there are no agent that causes the disease. The act will not only to pull hair strands away of the scalp, but the hairs that remain could split or turn frizzy. It is crucial to wait until your hair is dry to style and brush the hair. This aspect of the hair care routine is essential, especially since it helps prevent further loss of hair.

Avoid excessive stress. It is also essential to not put too much stress on yourself in the event of hair loss. Stress can affect the body so often that when it affects your life, a variety of signs of illness become evident. The loss of hair is not only an immediate symptom of stress, but also an indication of a condition that is caused by stress. Anything that is excessive will cause damage, and even more loss of excessive hair. Loss of hair can cause further damage to your health and wellbeing, which can cause further stress.

Do not attend too many salons. A lot of cutting and processing can weaken hair and lead to further loss of hair. It's a good idea to visit the salon frequently and have the professional haircuts, but be sure you allow your hair to get bigger and longer prior to making this trip. Let your hair grow by itself without the help of harmful chemicals and excessive styling. The best you can do is enrich the hair using homemade products that nourish and moisturize the scalp instead of using the harmful treatments at the salon which can tear hair strands off of the scalp.

Avoid excessive heating. Like we said earlier, avoid extreme treatments that involve high levels of chemical and heat. These could be offered by the salons one visits or even by curling and straightening irons, or hair dryers used daily. In the best way possible, or, if time permits let the hair dry naturally and choose simple haircuts that is managed quickly and effectively. If someone is experiencing continuous hair loss, keep away from hot hair dryers since they will surely cause the loss and thinning of the hair.

Do not suffer from dry, flaky scalp. Moisturize. Massage the scalp with essential oils that are natural to keep your scalp healthy. Healthy scalps mean healthy hair, as it assists in the growth and development of hair. It is important to select natural products to avoid to cause further harm to the scalp, and let it open for further injury. Remember that many natural remedies, like saw palmetto are able to combat hair loss as their extracts slow the development of DHT hormone, which is the cause of hair loss among men. These benefits are already beneficial in the reduction and prevention of loss of hair.

Don't wear hair wigs. The worst way to go if one suffers from a growing loss of hair is to wear the hairpiece. If the goal is to cover up the spots of baldness, you can do that, but it's not going to assist in stopping the reduction in hair. The wigs can only accelerate hair loss due to the heat they release and the pressure they put on the scalp. Patients who undergo radiation treatment who are experiencing hair loss may eventually cut off their hair in order to speed up the natural process of losing hair and make the process easier to wear a wig. It is recommended to address the root of the problem first, and then take preventive measures to stop the condition from getting worse.

Chapter 12: Hair Loss Cure

As of now, the science hasn't yet found the solution to complete hair loss. The most effective thing sufferers from hair loss and balding do is to increase the amount of hair has been left, to stimulate new hair growth and limit any further loss of hair.

It is a normal part of aging to experience hair loss. Hair loss that is excessive can be caused by environmental and genetic elements like diet and usage of products that contain harmful chemicals.

If you use all of the natural techniques which were covered in the previous chapters you're already reducing hair loss, and encouraging hair growth. If the natural approaches don't work, you'll have recourse to the recourse to prescription and over-the-counter medications.

Minoxidil is a popular medication for androgenetic alopecia. It is also known as pattern-baldness and alopecia areata which is the loss of hair caused by autoimmune issues. Minoxidil is available over-the-counter and prescriptionmedications, though the latter is more powerful. The treatment is available either in the form foam or liquid and is applied directly to the scalp. The hair growth resulting from minoxidil is likely to be less thick and won't last like normal hair, however it will conceal areas of hair loss. It should take about three months before the effects become evident.

Steroid hormones like corticosteroids are a different form that treat hair loss specifically the alopecia areata. It is injected into your scalp each month , or taken as a pill. Corticosteroids that are in the form of topical ointments can also be found but they aren't as efficient.

In the case of hair loss due to skin conditions like Psoriasis. Anthralin can be used to treat. The medication prescribed by a doctor is available in the form of an ointment that is applied on the scalp, causing the hair follicles in order to grow hair. It takes at least three months before the effects are evident.

For male pattern hair loss, the oral prescription Finasteride is a medication used. It aids in promoting hair growth by prolonging your anagen stage.

If none of the above options work then you could consider surgical options like hair transplants. Hair, and its roots are surgically removed from different parts of the body, or from a portion of the scalp, and transferred to the most prominently bald areas on the one side of your head. It can require several sessions before treatment is finished. It may also not always prove effective for all people.

Remember the fact that treatments like this should be used as a "last option." In the majority of cases changing your food and hygiene habits are sufficient to slow the loss of hair and help promote development of hair that is stronger.

Chapter 13: The Myths of Hair Loss

There's a lot of a man who is more hairy than his wit." - William Shakespeare

There are more myths than there are facts regarding hair loss. It is possible that they were born from desperation or to make a point that there is something wrong with them. Some might have some scientific foundation however some are plain funny. Let's look at the truth behind some of the most well-known hair myths.

The sun! It's burning!

It is widely accepted that exposure to the sun causes you bald, and ultraviolet (UV) Rays are the ones to blamed. This is not the case. Although UV rays can be blamed responsible for the accelerated aging process or skin cancer it will not affect the normal function of follicles. Don't avoid the sun like a plague. Wear your shades and go outdoors. Find a nice tan while enjoying yourself.

I'm not a shampoo person Thanks.

Sometimes we are tired to gaze down at the drain of our shower and find it blocked with hair that has fallen. We put the blame on shampoo. We conclude that it's not the proper formula, or is too strong and ought to use infant shampoo. If you're feeling like this then don't. It is possible to lose 100 hair strands every day. The majority of it is lost when you're bathing. It's part of the normal growth process. These hairs fall off and are replaced with new hairs that enter the anagen phase, also known as growth. Please stop crying about the follicles that have been dripping, well, hairs.

Oh! I'm getting older, and I'm balding.

It is believed that the loss of hair occurs with age. This is true, since genetic hair loss becomes more frequent as we get older, but it's not an all-encompassing issue. The most important thing to remember is that it doesn't care about age. The condition has been reported to be a problem for young people who are in their 20s and 30s. Because baldness caused by genetics can progress, the sooner you start to lose hair, the more severe it'll get, unless managed.

Let's look inside the hat that is magic... an encrusted small clump of hair!

It's believed to be the stressing of hair follicles which causes them to fall out. or the heat getting trappedand causing them to swell to death. Or the absence of oxygen flow to hair. Let's fix this. Caps and hats aren't the cause of the hair to fall out. They don't put enough stress or heat on hair to cause to be concerned. The hair isn't breathing. It is able to absorb oxygen from blood that flows through the scalp. The discussion is over.

Avoid sprays for hair and gels. They're the worst.

As with shampoo, styling products like gels mousse and sprays won't direct cause the loss of hair. However, if you use irons or tease the hair often, it is more prone to breakage or fallout. Be gentle with your hair, or you'll lose it in the near future.

Blame mom.

Researchers have discovered that the gene that is responsible for hair loss is located on the X chromosome that you inherit from your mother. This makes the hereditary cause stronger on the side of her. Research has shown that those with hair loss have a higher chance to become hair loss than those with no. Therefore, it's a 50-50 chance and don't show mom the look you'll get when you go to her with that piece of hair in your hands.

More sex, less hair.

As bizarre as it may be yet, this myth is an extremely well-known. The most fascinating theory is that the over-excessive ejection of seminal fluid can cause the deficiency of protein, which is the basis of hair. It makes sense If only there was an actual medical or scientific fact to support it. Excessive sex, or masturbation, doesn't cause hair loss. In the event that it is, everyone should be bald by the time they reach 30. Take a look at Hugh Hefner. He's still got hair, albeit it's gray, as it might be. He is the owner of the Playboy mansion. Can you imagine? Stop worrying and just enjoy yourself. Be safe.

Make the headstand.

Another of the most popular myths that is founded on the belief the fact that increased circulation of blood equals an increase in hair nutrients. But it's not so. If you sit on your head for too long you'll get dizzy, or your blood pressure could rise a bit but it doesn't at all, reverse loss of hair. Therefore, only do it during your yoga routine. Massages on the scalp aren't very harm either, since hair loss or retention don't actually depend on increased blood flow. It's a great way to relax isn't it? We need more of this I'd like to have more, please.

Chapter 14: Organic solutions to prevent hair loss

In this section you will discover solutions to stop hair loss. Keep in mind that, unlike medicines the natural solutions will solve your issue without causing any adverse side effects.

Oil massage

In the majority of instances hair loss is a result due to dry scalp and the hair follicles weak. If you perform a regular massage with various oils, you can keep your scalp moisturized and will assist in helping hair follicles grow stronger. A gentle massage will increase the circulation of the scalp which makes you feel calmer and less stressed.

There are a variety of oils that you could use for scalp massage such as coconut almond, castor, rosemary, amla argan, emu and wheat germ. The massage should be done with care, as excessive pressure could cause hair loss. The treatment is recommended to repeat every week at least in order to ensure the most effective outcomes.

Aloe vera

If you're in search of an effective natural solution to stop loss of hair, there's nothing better then aloe Vera. The benefits of applying Aloe Vera for your scalp is the growth of hair, a well-balanced pH, and reduction of itching on your scalp. Additionally, aloe vera may aid in restoring the natural shine and luster of their hair, making the roots healthier and removing scalp dandruff.

The most effective results can be achieved by using fresh aloe vera. However, it is also suggested to use the gel. The gel or juice of aloe vera should be applied directly to the scalp , and then left for about two hours. Once this natural treatment has performed its work, it is recommended to clean it off with warm water. The process is recommended to repeat every week.

Chinese hibiscus flower

It is believed that the Chinese have always provided the best solutions for a variety of medical conditions. The hibiscus plant that comes from Chinas is a potent source of benefits and can be used to prevent hair loss. It also stimulates the growth of hair by eliminating dandruff and assisting hair strands grow more dense.

If you're looking to combat hair loss using this remedy that is natural, mix the Chinese flowers of hibiscus with coconut oil. The mixture should be heated before being separated. After the remaining solution has cool then the next step will be applying the solution to hair. As with other natural remedies to combat loss of hair, it is best when left overnight. In the morning, shampoo your hair before applying conditioner. Repeat the process 2 or 3 times in a week.

Beetroot

Beetroot juice can be recommended as a natural remedy to prevent hair loss, specifically when the cause is deficiencies in vitamins or nutrients. The beneficial vitamins and nutrients found in beetroot can aid in making hair strands strongerand prevent hair loss.

There are two ways that beetroot juice could be utilized to help prevent hair loss. In the first scenario it is to take a sip of the juice and allow it work its magic. If you're keen on applying directly make sure you mix the beetroot leaves and henna then apply the mixture to your hair. Keep it on the hair for around a quarter hour, then wash it off using warm water. Repeat the process two or three times in a week.

Onions

Onions are regarded as a natural remedy for stopping hair loss since their juice is high in sulfur. There are two essential facts you need to know about onion juice. The first is that it helps improve scalp's blood circulation, and secondly, it helps in the regeneration of hair follicle. Additionally, due to its antibacterial properties, it helps to eliminate bacteria that cause hair loss.

If you're thinking about the benefits of this remedy that is natural, it is recommended to apply the juice of an onion directly on your scalp. To achieve the most effective results, allow it to sit for around 30 minutes, before washing it away by using warm water. Wash your hair, then apply conditioner. Another option is to mix the juice of an onion with olive oil and aloe vera doing the same process like the one mentioned above. The process should be carried out at least two to three every week until the first signs are evident.

Licorice root

If you're suffering from hair damage or hair loss, you should seriously consider using licorice root as a remedy that is natural. It will aid in eliminating hair loss and dandruff. It also helps in decreasing inflammation on the scalp and encouraging growth of hair.

The root of the licorice plant must be crushed and then mixed with saffron and milk. The paste is applied to hair (particularly on the areas that are bald) and then left for the night. The next day it is recommended to wash your hair in the same manner as you would normally. The treatment should be used every two or three days of the week for most effective results.

Fenugreek seeds

Fenugreeks seeds are a natural cure for a vast spectrum of illnesses, and are extremely effective when it comes to stopping or preventing hair loss. The active ingredients contained in Fenugreek seeds help to increase hair growth, as well as aiding the hair follicle to become stronger.

The suggestion is to soak the seeds of fenugreek in water, to soften them. Once they are soft they can be incorporated into the form of a paste. The paste is then applied to hair, and left for approximately 30 minutes. The process will be completed by a rinse of warm water. In order for the benefits of fenugreek seeds evident, this treatment should be used for a full month, starting every morning.

Flaxseeds

The fatty acids in flaxseeds makes them the ideal natural cure for loss of hair. Furthermore, this remedy helps to promote hair growth. If you'd like to take advantage of the properties of flaxseeds, you should include them in your diet. They can be eaten ground or directly added to other food items, like salads. It is also possible to apply them topically Flaxseed oil is advised as a natural remedy for hair loss.

Indian gooseberry

The plant is also referred to as amla and is well-known for its health benefits. If you're looking to prevent hair loss, it is a must to consider this natural solution. It is rich in vitamin C it could aid in maintaining hair health and will also help to increase hair growth.

To get the most effective results For the best results, mix the pulp of this fruit together with lemon juice freshly squeezed. Then, apply the mixture on their hair by giving it gentle massage. To achieve the best results, you may prefer to keep this treatment for your hair through the next day. The next day, wash your hair and use conditioner for your hair.

Potato juice

The juice of potatoes is suggested as a natural remedy to prevent hair loss because it is a rich source of vitamins (A B, C and A). If you're looking to try this remedy that is natural, make gratings of a few potatoes, then squeeze out the juice. Apply the juice of the potato directly on your scalp, and leave it for about a quarter of an hour. Rinse off the scalp with warm water. Repeat the procedure two to every three days.

A natural alternative to this cure is to mix potato juice , egg yolks and honey. The resultant mixture is applied to the hair and left on for about an hour and a half. A water rinse may suffice to remove the mix from hair therefore, make sure to wash it off afterwards. This option is recommended particularly those suffering with dry scalp. It will provide the right amount of moisture in order to prevent hair loss.

Eggs

Eggs are a rich source of proteins, making them extremely effective as a natural remedy for hair loss. It is possible to mix eggs yolks together with olive oil before applying it directly on the hair. Rinse off the mixture with warm water, and repeat the process two to three times per week.

The egg white can be utilized for a home remedy for hair loss. To get the most effective results egg whites should be mixed with honey and olive oil. The resultant mixture must be applied to hair and left for at least a quarter hour. Since the mixture is extremely dense, it is suggested to wash it off by shampoo.

Beetroot

Beetroot juice can be recommended as a natural remedy to prevent hair loss, particularly in cases where the issue is due to deficiencies in vitamins or nutrients.

The beneficial vitamins and nutrients that are present in beetroot help to make the hair strands more resilient, and will prevent loss of hair.

There are two ways that beetroot juice could be utilized to stop loss of hair. In the first case it is to consume the juice and let it work its work. If you're looking to apply it directly make sure you mix henna and beetroot leaves then apply the mixture to your hair. Apply it to the scalp for around a quarter hour, then wash it off using warm water. Repeat the process two or three times in a week.

Coconut milk

The protein and fats found in coconut milk may aid in stopping the loss of hair. They also help to promote the growth and growth of hair. If you are using freshly-made coconut milk as well as the commercial type, ensure that it is applied directly on the scalp and keep it for around 20 minutes. Shampoo and then apply conditioner.

A different option is to mix coconut milk with ground black pepper, and Fenugreek seeds. The mixture should put directly onto hair, then rinsed off. Both treatments should be repeated at least three times per week to get the most effective results.

Hot pepper

The main substance in peppers that is hot is called capsaicin making them a fantastic solution to stop hair loss. Capsaicin supplements, which are made by grinding hot peppers, can boost hair growth and will prevent the loss of existing hair. Hot peppers is consumed in its entirety with all the health-promoting qualities mentioned above.

Apple cider vinegar

If you're looking for an organic remedy to stop hair loss while also promoting growing hair as well as stimulating hair follicles you've come to the right place. It is suggested because it may improve the pH of scalp. If you are planning to use it as a remedy for your scalp ensure that you mix it with water , and then apply it to your scalp. For best outcomes, add an essential oil (lavender for instance) to the mix. Remember that applying the vinegar in its undiluted form can result in burns.

Neem (Indian Lilac)

Herbs like Neem have been utilized for centuries to increase hair growth and prevent loss of hair. If you are also suffering from dandruff, this is the ideal solution for you. The treatment is easy to follow: simmer the Neem leaves, then strain them. Apply the solution on the hair and wash it by using warm water. Repeat this process 2 or 3 times in a week.

Curd

Curd is natural treatment for loss of hair, and also to promote hair growth simultaneously. It can be used along with honey or black pepper. The resultant mixture should be applied to hair. The honey mixture is recommended for people suffering with dry scalp as it helps keep the scalp hydrated and keep hair loss. The mixture should be used for a quarter hour, and then washed by using warm water.

Garlic

Garlic is a potent herb with many benefits and is recommended as a natural remedy to prevent hair loss, especially when you have an illness brought on by an infection. To get the most effective results, garlic must be cooked in coconut oil. The resultant mixture should be allowed to cool before being applied to the hair. A gentle massage of the scalp can facilitate an even distribution of mixture. After the application, the hair needs to be shampooed. This process is recommended to repeat the process two or three times per week.

Black pepper and lemon juice

It is an acidic juice, and it can be a powerful natural remedy for losing hair by balancing the pH of scalp. To get the most effective results, it is suggested that lemon juice freshly squeezed is blended with grounded black pepper. The mixture is applied directly on the scalp, and kept for about a quarter of an hour. After that, it needs to be washed off using warm water. The process is repeated at least once a week.

Chapter 15: Natural Treatment

Hair loss treatments that are natural can also be found. They don't need the use of medication to boost hair growth or for surgery. They are also with a lower cost and is safer. The best part is that some can be found in your own backyard or in your kitchen pantry.

There are solutions that will require only to alter your routine or diet. Certain hair loss can be caused by stress or unhealthy lifestyles. Here are some natural hair treatment that you can use to encourage growth of your hair.

Exercise

Exercise improves blood circulation all across the body. It may aid with hair growth stimulation because hair follicles are stimulated to grow hair once more.

Herbs

There are many herbs that can assist you with the loss of hair. They are typically applied to the scalp that is affected. The hair loss you experience is dependent on your situation, the effects of each herb differs.

* Cassia Auriculata or Senna or Tanner Cassia is one of the most important ingredients in a variety of hair products. It helps to increase hair growth by stimulating the flow of blood throughout the scalp. It also functions as a antibacterial and tonic that helps treat scalp issues. This helps to promote shiny and thick hair.

* Hibiscus Rosa-Sinensis is also known by its name of China rose. It is believed to increase hair growth. It is a healing flower it helps prevent hair loss or premature graying. It also aids in treating hair loss and scalp conditions.

* Henna or Mehandi is well-known to cleanse, color and condition hair. It was used for centuries by royalty and also provides the hair a shiny, glossy finish. It soothes the scalp, decreases hair fall and adds volume to the hair.

* Curry leaves are popular for adding flavor to food items, but they also provide a great treatment for hair. It replenishes hair and helps strengthen hair follicles. It also aids in hair growth because it functions as an antioxidant.

* Chrysopogon Zizaniodes is a plant that improves circulation and helps nourish the shaft of hair.

* Rose petals are used to soothe and nourish the hair. They remove flaky skin, and also increases blood flow, which decreases hair loss and increases hair volume.

* Neem is a remedy for hair loss because it promotes hair growth. It contains fatty acids, which help to promote healthy hair

growth and has been utilized for hundreds of years.

Nutrition

Nutrition plays a significant part in promoting hair growth, but it is also important to stop hair loss. If you're looking to be healthier and better it is important to be aware of the food you consume.

Protein is crucial in stimulating hair growth. It stimulates hair growth, which is why it's advised to consume 2 to 3 servings of dairy, meat and beans, which is around 3 pounds daily.

Omega-3 rich foods are also essential to include in your diet. These are discovered in nuts, seeds as well as fish. This reduces inflammation and helps to promote a healthy scalps.

The iron supplement is suggested to reduce your risk for anemia that is one of the primary reasons for hair loss. It also helps improve circulation of blood, which stimulates growth of hair.

* Vitamin C aids in iron absorption. It is found in food items like strawberries, oranges and grapes.

Biotin and zinc help to promote hair growth, particularly for those suffering from metabolic disorders.

Treatment for Hair Loss

When you go through an operation or home remedy for your loss of hair, you should be sure to include an appropriate diet. Examine your diet and ensure that you prepare your own healthy menu. Make sure you are familiar with the right foods that contain the nutrients you require to maintain healthy hair.

Chapter 16: Different types of shampoos and conditioners

Shampoos come with very similar components like preservatives, surfactants and foam enhancers and scents frequently however the variations in the healing and caring ingredients create a range of different types of shampoo.

Shampoos designed for normal hair make up the most extensive category of shampoossince they are recommended for those with hair that is healthy. This category includes all neutral or acid-balanced shampoos. Shampoos that are of high-quality do not have an alkaline pH, but do contain minimal components necessary for hairstyling and are a typical mix of cleansing elements. The primary function of these shampoos is washing the hair while maintaining the health and appearance of hair. These shampoos are generally not advised for daily use.

Hair shampoos that are dry. Dry hair looks like straw and splits at the ends. It's stubborn all season. The ideal product for hair that is dry has elements for hydration that aids in reducing dryness. Shampoo that contains different oils or butters is perfect for this type of hair.

Hair shampoos that are suitable for those with oily. In general the hair that is oily (due to an excessive production of sebum) is stale when washed almost immediately. This is particularly true for hair that is located near the scalp. A good Shampoo for hair with oily flakes needs to comprise ingredients like essential oils and plant extracts which help restore the normal production of sebum.

Shampoos for hair with color are part of the specific category of hair color which is designed to maintain the color of the hair. They have mild components that do not wash away the color of the hair. The formula of shampoos for hair that is colored always comprises creams, emollients and silicone Emulsions. In this situation the shampoo formula suggests the use of shampoos and conditioners that improve the effectiveness of keeping the color. But, if your hair is lightened, chemically curled, straightened, or dyed, this kind of shampoo will not aid; it does not have the ability to regenerate your hair. If this is the case it is recommended to take note of shampoos specifically designed that treat damaged hair.

The shampoo that is designed for hair damage kind of shampoo that restores the hair's structure after damage and gives it look and feel of hair that is healthy. Its purpose is to cleanse delicately damaged scalps and hair without causing any further damage. In addition it helps to increase the volume of hair by smoothing the surface. The category of damaged hair comprises hair that has been damaged through repeated lightening, coloring and chemical treatments to alter the shape of hair (perm and straightening) as well as intense temperature exposure and aggressive combing. Hair that is damaged like this is typically rough and fragile, and not able to hold cosmetic color due to severe injury to the cuticle as well as cortex layers.

The moisturizing shampoos are designed to treat dry hair. The aim for moisturizing shampoos are fill and retain moisture in hair. They contain a huge variety of conditioning agents hence they are often called conditioning shampoos. They contain moisturizing and emollient fats and oils, like lecithin, lanolin oil, argan oil Jojoba, and a few others. They possess a mild antistatic effect and help improve hair handling. It is not recommended to apply moisturizing shampoos in cases of thin hair or oily hair roots.

The category of medicated shampoos comprises an entire range of products made of unique medicinal ingredients to treat issues with the scalp. Shampoos to treat dandruff, shampoos treating seborrhea, shampoos for sensitive scalp as well as shampoos for hair loss fall in this category. In most cases, for the intricate treatment of of these issues there are a variety of therapeutic agents, the most notable that is shampoo. The most notable feature of dandruff shampoos is their ability to combat the fungus responsible for causing the dandruff. Sometimes, dandruff doesn't result from of fungus however, it is due to dry skin (mainly the season). In such instances the application of moisturizing products is suggested. If after a period of 2-3 weeks of using dandruff shampoo and dandruff is still not gone consult a trichologist for consultation. Shampoos designed for oily hair (shampoos for treating seborrhea) generally contain proper cleansing ingredients that are medicated, but have no effects on conditioning. The formula of the shampoo has unique components that provide antimicrobial effects and can decrease the production of sebum on the scalp. The medicated shampoos are acidic pH as the alkaline environment boosts sebum production. But, oily and dandruff hair shampoos are both strong cleansing properties, which is why the color of the hair is thoroughly removed from the color hair. Shampoos for scalps with sensitive skin is another type of shampoos that are therapeutic. It is a must-have drug for those who find that each wash can cause irritation and itching. Shampoos designed for sensitive scalps tend to be very gentle and won't cause irritation to the scalp. They contain a wide range of componentsthat reduce the impact on the scalp. They also contain natural remedies to relieve irritation to the skin. Shampoos that treat hair loss are typically the most gentle of all shampoos that contain medicated ingredients. They are made with the softest ingredients within their formulation. The main functions of this shampoo is to cleanse the scalp of harmful substances with ease as well as to nourish the skin with nourishment and prepare it for the next stage of treatment.

In certain instances shampoos may have an impact on the skin since they are just one of the initial steps in treatment. Skin irritation is the reason for the fast absorption of therapeutic drops, lotions and masks that are applied following shampoo. All the subsequent drugs are sedative which means they ease irritation. Be aware that shampoo for hair loss won't be able to heal by itself, without further procedures and can cause irritation the scalp and, in some instances, cause itching and burning.

Shampoos designed for hair with hair that is thin (volumizing shampoo) provide a look that increases the size of the hair. These shampoos are made up of a vast variety of polymer compound (membrane-forming chemicals) and silicones. These create a thin, slightly rough skin on the hair's surface to create the appearance of volume. The membrane lasts only a few days, since it's washed off in part after shampooing. But, with the regular use of shampoo to increase the volume, one must be aware of the cumulative effects and cleanse the hair with an intensely cleansing shampoo.

Curly Hair Shampoos. The curly hair type is more porous as well as brittle due to the fact that its core is curled by nature. Shampoos for curly hair need to be gentler than regular shampoos hair because it is more susceptible to dryness, particularly if colored. Make sure to use products that have a high percentage of different oils that improve the health of the hair on the inside and aid in maintaining a healthy moisture level. You can also use a special shampoos specifically designed for curly hair.

Coloring shampoos are an extremely popular option for coloring hair, increasing the colorand neutralizing undesirable shades. This line includes very popular shampoos that conceal gray hair, as well as shampoos for women with hair colored in blond , anti-yellow shampoos and shampoos which enhance the brown and red hair. Colored shampoos are the usual shampoos for colored or natural hair with one feature that is the presence of colored pigments that add hair color when washed. These shampoos won't cause damage to hair and won't make hair lighter, since they do not contain alkaline or oxygenizing ingredients. They simply add or alter the shade of hair. The resultant shade isn't lasting and can be washed away using regular shampoo. It is possible to create an unattractive coloration on extremely blonde hair after applying coloring shampoo. In this instance shampoo should be applied slowly, and possibly diluting water. It is based on the porosity of hair.

The deep cleaning shampoos offer distinct, primarily salon-style variant of shampoos. The principal function of deep cleansing shampoos is to get rid of all the build-up of hair by styling and washing. The shampoo is extremely powerful cleansing components. This is why it should be recommended only when there's visible accumulation on hair, and not more less than twice a week. It treats scalp and hair effectively, and is able to wash away the hair's color quickly and does not require the application of a conditioner following the wash. It may cause dryness and irritation of the skin, dandruff and dry hair when it is used regularly. use. It's NOT recommended that you use a strong cleaning shampoo for home use. shampoo.

Shampoos designed for everyday use are typically gentle shampoos designed for normal hair and are suitable for use on a daily basis. They generally come with an acidic pH as well as a cleanser ingredients that are non-irritating.

Dry shampoos (waterless shampoos) are used in situations where it's difficult washing your hair using regular shampoo. Dry shampoos come in two forms which are spray and powder. The shampoos consist of mild alkali and starch in their composition. Alkali converts sebum into soap, while the starch absorbs dirt, oil and then the soap that results. The remainder part of shampoo gets eliminated by combs. It is to be aware that dry shampoos add volume hair, but they can be hard to manage and can cause dry hair to dry. The alkali shows the cuticle's scales layer, and they aren't able to close. Be cautious when styling your hair that has been washed using dry shampoo.

Universal 2-in-1 shampoo one of a set of shampoos that combine conditioning shampoo as well as conditioner. They do not require the use of conditioners and masks since they're responsible for washing and smoothing out the cuticle of hair. For a better outcome, you should use shampoo and conditioner in a separate manner. Since the majority of shampoos cleanse hair, and conditioners contain ingredients which nourish and protect hair.

Baby shampoos are typically gentle cleanser that won't cause irritation to the eyes. They typically contain the most gentle cleanser ingredients, along with conditioning ingredients. Because children are less likely to produce sebum as adults do, this kind of shampoo is not suitable for people who are adults. It is difficult for baby shampoo to deal with the level of hair buildup.

If you're satisfied with your shampoo routine and it's not harmful to your hair, you are able to keep using it. However, if you aren't choose to go with products that contain natural ingredients. The shampoo is made from oil, medicinal plants as well as vitamins and nutrients. The best shampoos are made up of many ingredients. Be sure to look for organic shampoos.

Organic shampoos don't build up toxic substances within the epidermis layer and do not break the natural lipid barrier unlike products containing sulfate. Sulfate shampoos quickly remove color, whereas natural products, on contrary, maintain the color. This happens because organic shampoos do not ruffle the hair's scales and the color stays in your hair for longer duration.

The major distinction in regular and organic versions is the raw ingredients. Thus, the formulation of organic shampoo ought to include 95% of organic and natural ingredients. There aren't any such requirements for the production of normal shampoos, and most of the time, the label concentrates on these or other natural ingredients that make up the product could be lower than one percent. So, it's important to check the label and , in particular the composition prior to purchasing. Most organic shampoos don't contain SLS. The organic shampoo's consistency is more fluid than regular shampoos since they do not contain thickeners or natural ones and transparent without glossy shine and have a sour typically subtle scent. They aren't sucked up well since they have gentle cleansing ingredients. Thus, even in the absence of foam that is rich the shampoo is able to cleanse your hair well. It is important to note that organic shampoos aren't made to be used regularly or on a daily basis.

Conditioners. Shampoos are used to get rid of sebum, residues from styling products dead skin cells and dirt from scalp hair. The cuticle, which typically protects the hair shaft in an equally thick layer, shifts little bit off from hair's shaft following washing. In this instance hair shafts are more prone to damage impacts of the environment as well as extreme temperatures. This is why conditioners. They return the cuticle back to its original position and they secure it to the hair shaft. The hair is now ready for styling and is able to take on the pressures of daily life without causing damage. Hair will become more accommodating and retains moisture, giving shine to the hair following the application of conditioner.

In general, conditioners are best applied throughout the length of hair. Avoid applying conditioner to the scalp or the hair's roots as the hair's volume will decrease and appear dirty in this region; conditioning can cause skin dryness and lead to the scalp to itch or cause hair loss due to dandruff. Apply a tiny amount on the hair and distribute it along all the length with a combing comb using the rare teeth.

It is recommended for people who have hair that is oily to use conditioner only to the ends of hair.

When you've applied the conditioning it is essential to rinse it off within some time so that it is able to penetrate the cuticle. It is also recommended to dry your hair prior to applying the conditioner in order to get rid of moisture and maximize effectiveness.

Chapter 17: Factors influencing hair quality

Hair acts as an exterior cover for the scalp, and is regularly exposed to the external environment. In general, the weather impacts the hair's chemical structure as UV radiation, humidity winds, pollutants, and humidity affect hair and can cause a hair loss and a poor texture. The variation in regional hair quality is notable because of the effect of weather. Weather is an important factorthat is evident in the country-wise loss of hair phenomenon. Hair damage caused by weather is more prevalent among Asian and Caucasian people, while harsh chemical-induced hair damage is common among African Americans, as they apply a lot of chemicals to the head to smooth the appearance of hair.

The hair's unique structure provides its own strength of resistance to stand up to the harshest weather conditions. Cuticle and cortex coatings form an outer layer of protection over hair that helps make it stronger. The 10% of the weight of hair is by the cuticles that cover it. The cuticles are placed in tiny scale-like forms that overhang each other, with the exposed edges are positioned towards the edges. Disulfide bonds are found in keratin. They strengthen hair by forming layers that are embedded within the structure of cortex. Additionally, melanin in the cortex offers protection to hair from UV radiation.

Free radicals are produced by the interaction of UV Rays, water and iron, and can cause damage to hair's photosynthesis. Melanin is a natural antioxidant that is able to neutralize free radicals as well as take in UV radiation. However, excessive exposure UV radiation could degrade melanin. In time, the protein structures found in hair cross-link to form a the cortex structure. The result of this biological modification of hair causes them to become fragile. Photodamage is more prevalent when people have a blond hair colors. Pheomelanin is the melanin that is found in hair with blond color that is less resistant in the face of UV radiation than the eumelanin. People with gray hair also suffer from similar issues due to changes in melanin composition.

The hair grooming routine and climate conditions contribute on hair growth and hair damage. The effects isn't always immediate but the results are noticeable in the hair loss due to age. The smooth cuticle is a source of shining, healthy looking hair. The roughness of hair is due to the properties of friction in cuticle and is observable through the combing process or when touching the hair. Hair that is splotchy, which is clinically known as trichoptilosis, is a typical problem among long hair, which is often exposed in the sun's UV radiation.

The control of climate conditions isn't within our control. Hair grooming is an crucial to loss of hair. Thus, regular hair grooming will help reduce damage to hair even in the harshest weather. Here are some suggestions to ensure a healthy and safe hair grooming routine:

Make use of mild shampoos to clean your hair since it is antiseptic and soothes your scalp that also provides moisture to your hair.

Massaging the scalp and hair during shampooing, improves circulation and assists with hair growth.

• Avoid frequent perming of your hair.

Avoid permanent hair dye.

Hair beaching frequently is not a good hair grooming routine.

Always brush dry hair from the scalp until the ends.

Make sure to use a broad-toothed or a round brush for a more gentle combing.

The frequent drying of hair is not recommended, because it causes hair to dry out and causes it to become more fragile. [6]

The diagnosis of hair loss

Because hair loss is often due to a myriad of causes, it is crucial to identify the root cause in order to pinpoint the root of the hair loss. This can assist in determining the most effective treatment to treat the problem by resolving the causes. A blood test specific to the condition can be conducted to identify any hormonal imbalance or thyroid diseases, or the beginning of cancer. A dermatologist may conduct a pull test order to determine the amount of loss of hair by gently pulling your hair. The test will also help determine the degree of loss. Microscopy using light is an exam to examine the health of the hair's roots of the hair, as well as to identify any anomalies on the hair's root. A scalp biopsy could be taken in the event of an unexpected significant loss of hair and to identify any metastatic growth or infection that is affecting the hair's roots. [7]

Reducing hair loss naturally

Hair loss isn't fatal. Thus, treating the condition by using synthetic medicines is not the best option. Since this could increase the amount of chemicals within the body. Minoxidil is among the most frequently prescribed medicines for treating hair loss. The Mayo clinic outlines potential adverse reactions that could be triggered by Minoxidil treatment. The most common side effects include such as itching or skin rash to the face (most commonly reported adverse effect) as well as swelling, redness of the skin and inflammation of the hair root as well as facial hair growth. burning sensations at the top of the head. A few users have also complained of the appearance of blurred vision and lightheadedness headache, dizziness and chest pain. They also experienced rapid weight growth, palpitations and a feeling of tingling on the both legs. In this section we will go over various scientifically-proven natural treatments to treat hair loss.

Chapter 18: Tips For Choosing Essential Oils

Organic

This is typically one of the primary aspects you should look for before using the essential oil you purchase or using. Make sure you choose essential oils that are extracted from organically grown vegetables since they are free of pesticide residues that could be more harmful than beneficial for your scalp and hair.

The extraction process

This is another thing you must look into. Essential oils are generally "harvested" by seeds in extraction. The extraction method used isn't just important to the overall high-quality of oil, but for your own security as well. Here are the most common kinds of extractions for essential oils:

* Steam press

Steam pressing refers to the process of using steam to apply heat to extract essential oil. The steam travels through the materials to vaporize the volatile oils. The volatile oils then rise in the steam. The steam is stored in the chamber of condensation.

* Solvent pressed

The name implies that this method makes use of the use of a solvent, such as the hexane. The process keeps the natural scent of the plant however solvents like Hexane aren't always secure - they could harm the nervous system if they are used in excessive amounts.

* Cold-pressed

The majority of essential oil experts have identified this method to be the most effective way to extract essential oils because the oil isn't damaged like it would when it is heated. Cold-pressed oils are typically identified by its light-colored color and fresh smell - the scent of the seeds does not disappear during the process. Cold pressing , however, isn't appropriate for extracting all essential oil.

Beware of the use of synthetic scents

It is important to recognize the difference between synthetic scent oils that are created through a chemical extraction processes in comparison to pure essential oils. Although they may have the same scent or have the exact same smell in pure essential oils,, their properties for therapeutic purposes might not be exactly identical.

Risks and potential complications of Essential oils

The greatest risk with essential oils is the possibility of allergic reactions to skin or allergic. It is commonplace when a person applies an essential oil that is not diluted directly on the skin. It is therefore essential to always apply an oil carrier to reduce the amount. Allergies are more frequent for those with sensitive skin or allergies to essential oils.

An allergic reaction can be identified by the signs that are:

* Tissue narrowing or swelling of the tongue.

* Trouble breathing

* Flaming rashes

* Severe dermatitis

Signs of skin irritation are:

* The affected area may be red.

* A painful tingling sensation or burning

* Contact dermatitis

Essential oils are best used by adults and older teens topically for health of their hair. If you are planning to apply essential oils for your child, first check with their doctor to make sure the use is safe. To determine if there is irritation, first test only a small amount of mixture on a small portion of your face prior to application.

Applying Essential Oils to Your Hair

Since essential oils are generally extremely concentrated, you don't want to apply them to your hair directly. There are several methods to apply them to your hair in a safe manner:

Make a spray: Mix the essential oil that you want to apply with aloe Vera in an aerosol bottle. Spray your hair with your mixture all day. If you're out in the open, citrus essential oils won't be effective for this kind of application.

Create conditioner: It's easy; you just need to mix the essential oil you prefer with a carrier oil, such as coconut oil, and then rub it into your hair. Let it sit for an to 2 hours or more and then rinse it out.

Make pomade by combining your essential oil with carrier oil, and then beeswax you can make pomade, which is a tool which encourages hair growth when you fashion your hair.

Enhance your shampooby adding the drops of your favorite essential oil to your shampoo , so it's applied to your scalp and hair when you shampoo.

Preventive Oils to Care for Hair

To effectively massage hair and avoid allergic reaction, make sure to keep this base oil light you can. For this make these oils more diluted by using carrier oils such as peach kernel, apricot kernel, grapeseed, and Jojoba oil.

If you have coarse and thick Try using rich, nourishment oils such as olive, avocado rose hip, hemp sesame and evening primrose oils. Be sure to create an appropriate hydrating agent that is balanced by mixing a good amount of natural oils and the appropriate carrier oils.

For instance, mix 3 to 5 drops of preventive oil in a teaspoon, or 5ml of the base oil such as Jojoba oil.

Once you've diluted the preventive oils, apply it into your scalp and hair, and let it soak for at least one hour or up to a night. After that, wash your hair with your normal shampoo and allow your hair naturally dry.

To rinse your hair, add 10-15 drops of the oils in this final rinse. This will improve the condition of locks and the scalp. Add some drops of your own homemade shampoo to boost the effectiveness of your shampoo. Remember that the natural oils typically evaporate quickly , and therefore shouldn't be left out in the open.

Seeds for Hair Loss

I have already mentioned the possibility of utilize various seeds (I mentioned flaxseed, fenugreek as well as cumin) to combat hair loss. The next chapter will cover the topic of hair loss. I will reiterate some of the points, but a lot of the seeds are new to you.

Mustard seeds

Mustard seeds can be a boon to improve the health of your scalp and hair. The mustard oil is extracted from mustard seeds. Mustard oil is very rich in vitamin A which is a vital vitamin for hair regeneration and scalp nourishment.

It's also vital to increase collagen which is crucial to maintain the elasticity and health of hair strands. If you're struggling with weak and fragile hair, it's your time to rejoice because mustard seeds are loaded with calcium, protein Omega three and six fatty acids, and vitamin A and E , all that help strengthen your hair from the inside. Strong hair means less hair loss.

As mentioned earlier As we have mentioned earlier, Vitamin E is a powerful antioxidant that can aid in the elimination of free radicals that build up in your scalp. This is one of the primary causes of loss of hair. It is good to know that the mustard seeds are brimming in vitamin E. the fatty acids contained in the oils extracted from seeds improves the condition and gives life to dull hair.

The oil also has B vitamins that aid in controlling the production of sebaceous glands, and helps to provide your hair with a gorgeous shine. The large amount of ALA and euric acids in the mustard oil is well-known for their ability to eliminate fungus naturally that is the primary cause of dry , itchy flake and hair dandruff.

Black seeds

They are among the most effective treatments to grow thicker hair and stopping loss of hair. They are helpful for different kinds of hair loss such as Alopecia, telogen effluxuim female pattern baldness as well as male pattern hair loss. Its botanical title is called nigella Sativa however it is also known under other names, including:

* Shuneiz,

* Fennel flower

* Black caraway

* Onion seeds

* Kalonji seeds

* Nutmeg flower

* Roman coriander

* Black cumin

Black seeds are a potent source of antioxidants that help to strengthen hair follicles as well as encouraging growth. The antioxidants assist by protecting the hair's cells against ageing process that thins the hair.

These seeds have another powerful compound called Thymoquinone (TQ) that is an anti-inflammatory compound that can stop the loss of hair caused by irritation of the hair follicles e.g. Alopecia and TE. The normal growth of hair is also achieved through the diminution of inflammation.

They also have nigellone, as well as other antihistamine ingredients that have been discovered to bring dormant hair follicles into a growth phase, which increases the quantity of hair on your scalp. The antihistamine can also aid in making hair's strands stronger.

The seeds are high of B Vitamins and Minerals like copper, zinc, and iron. These seeds are great for nourishing your hair. The fatty acids found in the seeds can also reduce dryness on the scalp and increase appearance and condition of hair.

Fenugreek seeds

I'm sure I've mentioned it previously, but I'll cover the subject from a different angle, I promise.

Fenugreek is used for a considerable period of time to treat ailments that cause dry, irritated skin, which includes dandruff. It is an irritant that is manifested by the scalp becoming itchy and flaking.

In certain instances the symptoms may result in temporary loss of hair. Dandruff can result from many diverse causes, such as dry skin and inflammation, as well as excessive oil production. It's unclear whether these seeds are able to help treat all the causes of scalp irritation or dandruff, but tests on animals and in test tubes show that they have wound healing skin soothing moisturizing, antifungal, as well as anti-inflammatory qualities. In a six-week study on the effectiveness of a cream that reduces the appearance of redness on the skin and improving the moisture of the skin using fenugreek extract as one of the ingredients eleven subjects showed significant improvement in the appearance of skin irritation as well as the amount of moisture.

Recent research suggests that application of the extracts of fenugreek may aid in maintaining healthy scalp. It is however not 100% certain that it will be effective for all who try it. It is necessary to conduct additional research on humans to gain a greater understanding of how this extract can be used to treat for dandruff as well as other scalp irritation.

You can consume the seeds orally in as a supplement to your diet or use it on your hair using masks and pastes. The supplements are sold as in a concentrated liquid extract, or in a powder form. There's no particular recommendation regarding dosage for oral use, however some research has suggested the consumption of extracts of 300 mg or 1200 milligrams of seed powder per every day. While it's generally safe for most individuals, you should steer clear of the supplements if you're allergic to peanuts or chickpeas or if expecting. If you're unsure you are allergic, consult your doctor.

Jojoba oil

Jojoba oil is an oil-like substance that is extracted from seeds of the Jojoba plant. It's employed as a moisturizer as it is an oily substance and can also be utilized as a treatment for hair dandruff. It can be added to your conditioner for extra protection against breakage, split ends and dryness.

The oil is also believed to increase hair's thickness and stop hair loss since it helps strengthen hair. The reasoning behind this is that because it moisturizes hair follicles, it helps prevent dryness which leads to hair loss.

Jojoba is abundant in vitamins and minerals that nourish hair, including zinc copper vitamin E, B vitamins , and Vitamin C.

Apply directly. Apply the oil directly to hair over the scalp, then gradually work it down to the hair's tips. Do not apply directly to the scalp to prevent the scalp from getting clogged pores. If you're applying the oil to treat dry scalp or dandruff apply about 1-2 drops directly onto the skin.

Find items that contain it. This is the most efficient method of getting and using the oil of jojoba. You can purchase natural conditioners or shampoo that contains Jojoba oil among the ingredients.

Include it in the products. It's easy to do to add three drops of Jojoba Oil into a tablespoon of your favorite conditioner , or shampoo prior to using it.

Flaxseeds

I'm sure I've mentioned the subject before but, as promised I'll add an entirely new perspective.

Flaxseeds are extremely beneficial for promoting hair growth as well as general well-being. Actually, flax is classified as a species called Usitatissimum which literally signifies "most beneficial".

They're a fantastic food source for Vitamin E which aids in enhancing the effectiveness of blood capillaries and improving circulation. Additionally, it has powerful antioxidants that protect against hair loss and scalp damage. Vitamin E is also helpful in preventing premature graying.

Alongside the vitamin E , flaxseeds are also high in omega-3 fatty acids, which are essential for the development in healthy hair. They feed hair shafts as well as hair follicles strengthening them and less prone to being damaged. This also ensures that the new hairs are healthy and sturdy. Omega 3 fatty acids aid in enhancing the hair's elasticity.

They also aid in controlling the production of oil and in balancing pH levels. Both of these factors directly impact the condition of your hair and the speed that it grows. They are a soothing effect on the scalp. They also assist in relaxing the sebaceous glands , ensuring they can produce the right amount of oil needed to grow hair.

Additionally, flaxseeds aid in soothing your scalp and conditioning hair. Regular use of flaxseeds , or even ingestion helps prevent problems like dandruff, scalp eczema, and severe hair loss. Apart from applying the seeds as an applied treatment for the skin, eating the seeds could also benefit your overall hair growth. They also are a fantastic source of both soluble and insoluble fibers. When it comes to improving the condition of your hair and hair shaft, flaxseeds aid with making hair smooth and manageable because they bind moisture into the shaft of your hair, thereby helping to control dryness, frizz split ends, breakage and split ends.

Here are a few methods to incorporate flaxseeds in your diet to boost your hair growth:

Grinding flaxseeds to a fine powder is a great way to include them in your diet. Incorporate the powder into your oatmeal, soup and muffins, milk or smoothies. Add it to cookies, smoothies, and muffins. The powder can be stored in an airtight container in the refrigerator.

* You could also consider adding flaxseeds in raw form to your diet, as it's one of the easiest methods. It is possible to sprinkle a teaspoon over stir-fried vegetables or salads to increase the taste while reaping the benefits of health.

Pumpkin seeds

Pumpkin seeds contain a compound called beta-sitosterol. It hinders the enzyme known as 5-alphareductase which converts testosterone into dihydrotestostetone (DHT). The excess of DHT within the body triggers male pattern baldness as well as hair loss through attachment to hair follicles resulting in the reduction of the growth phase.

Additionally, the seeds contain a chemical known as delta-7-sterine. It also is a competitor to DHT at receptor sites throughout the body.

Additionally, pumpkin seeds contain the highest levels of antioxidants essential fatty acids zinc and magnesium, which are, as we have discussed earlier help to promote hair growth.

Use: You could try including pumpkin seeds in your diet routine or rub oil taken from the seeds onto your scalp before going to going to bed. The idea is to let the essential omega-sitosterol, fatty acids, delta-7-sterine, and other ingredients in the seeds affect the hair follicles in the night.

It is also possible to take pumpkin seed oil, which comes typically in the form of capsules with oil gel. Be sure to follow the instructions on the label of the product you purchase. The typical dose is 1000 mg per capsule. It is possible to take one or 2 capsules by mouth after meals three times a every day. Because supplements aren't regulated by the FDA dosage and quality can differ, so make sure that you buy the products from reliable businesses for your personal safety. Stop taking supplements as soon as you are experiencing stomach pain or signs of food allergy. Always consult your doctor before use.

Chia seeds

Hair and chia seeds share one common element they share, protein. According to the book in the past, our hair is typically made of a protein called Keratin. However, chia seeds have approximately 23 percent protein. Therefore, you don't just receive fiber from seeds, but also their protein also, which help to strengthen your hair. Protein is essential to the growth and health of hair. Inadequate enough protein in your diet may cause hair growth in sows or even loss of hair.

Chia seeds are an excellent supply of B vitamins, specifically Niacin (vitamin B3) and Thiamin (vitamin B1) However, they also have additional B vitamins, including cobalamin (vitamin B12) and Pyridoxine (vitamin B6)) and of riboflavin (vitamin B2) in smaller quantities. According to numerous research studies, your body needs a sufficient amount of B complex vitamins to maintain healthy hair.

Chia seeds are a great source of iron from food. The majority of iron that you have in your body is located in hemoglobin, an amino acid that transports oxygen to your scalp and hair. So, it's obvious that it's vital for you to get enough iron to maintain healthy hair. Actually one of the major reasons for premature loss of hair loss in women is believed to be the depletion of iron stores.

Chia seeds are a great source of zinc and copper. While copper is required in small amounts within the body, it is essential for proper functioning and good hair growth. A lack of copper consumption in your daily diet is associated with hair loss, thinning and loss. It has also been believed to enhance hair's color and slow the it from graying. Zinc is an additional mineral that is essential to maintain healthy hair. Chia seeds are rich in zinc which plays an important role in the growth of hair growth and assists in controlling the production of oil. This gives your hair a shiny , glossy appearance.

Chia seed is a great natural source of alpha-linolenic acids (ALA) which is an essential omega-3 fatty acid which plays a vital role in all functions within the human body, including scalp and hair. Hair loss and scaly skin have been linked to an insufficient level of alpha linolenic acid as well as the linoleic acid.

Chapter 19: The Causes of Hair Loss

Hair loss is not a requirement mean that someone is suffering from a health issue. In some instances, the loss of the hair might be a normal part of the ageing process for the individual. However, alopecia could be caused by different causes that are not related to aging.

Factors that are responsible for hair loss

1. Genetics

It has been discovered that heredity is among the main causes of the majority of cases of alopecia. If a relative of the line, or any of your paternal or maternal relatives suffer from hair loss, it is likely that the genetics could be passed down to subsequent generations, which makes you more susceptible to suffer from hair loss also.

2. Autoimmune Disorders and other Medical Conditions

A specific autoimmune condition referred by the name of alopecia areata is believed to be one of the main causes of hair loss in people. With this condition your body's immunity can be found to alter hair follicles and, consequently creating hair loss in patches that are round and bald.

Apart from certain kinds of autoimmune conditions, other diseases and medical conditions can cause hair loss. This includes but is not restricted to the following thyroid diseases as well as skin and scalp infections and shingles, endocrine system issues, syphilis, as well as leprosy.

3. Medicines

Different kinds of medications utilized to treat ailments like depression, cancer as well as high blood pressure heart problems and gout are recognized for their adverse effects, including hair loss.

4. Hormonal imbalance

Alterations or imbalances in hormones in the body can cause the loss of hair for a short period. For women, loss of hair can occur as due to pregnancy and menopausal symptoms, birth, and the stopping of birth medication to control the birth.

5. Physical and emotional stress

Stress, whether emotional or physical, that is felt by the body is thought to result in hair loss too. Some examples of this include the stress that an individual experiences following a major operation, an extreme disease, or after a major problem or situations that can result in emotional stress as well as trauma (e.g. an accident).

To the energy to fixing the essential aspects of the body that are affected by emotional or physical tension, our body is prone to temporarily shut down activities and functions that aren't considered essential for survival. this includes hair production.

In addition to the factors mentioned earlier, additional factors that can cause hair loss are certain hairstyling methods, products and therapies, nutrition deficiencies and a specific disorder known as the disorder of pulling hair.

Understanding the root of the loss of hair in a person is essential to ensure that the issue can be dealt with in the most effective and most efficient manner possible.

Chapter 20: Hair Loss Prevention

"Prevention is better than curing.'

In fact, this statement has an abundance of truth in each and every word. Making proactive efforts to take good care of your hair when it's in its lush and full condition can make much in preventing loss of hair.

Prevention of hair loss does not require fancy tricks to be accomplished efficiently. Instead, it will require a few simple methods that you can implement into your everyday life and routines.

What to Make Your Hair Look After Your Hair

Excellent Hair Care Tips to Prevent Hair Loss

A well-balanced diet is essential, particularly foods that are high in vitamins like A B, C, iron, E and protein.

Comb or brush your hair with care and make sure to use combs with wide teeth whenever you can.

Make sure to use gentle and mild shampoos to wash your hair.

Do not apply extreme temperatures to your hair, like with hair straighteners or hair dryers because these items could cause damage to your hair, making it more brittle.

* Try to stay away from anxiety as far as you can since stress can contribute to the development of certain types of hair loss in addition to how it may cause negative effects on general health.

Apply a massage to your hair with the essential oils every now and then.

Drink plenty of fluids.

Reduce your consumption of alcohol.

* Stop smoking.

* Make sure that your body is getting the right quantity of workout.

Be careful not to comb your hair when it is still damp.

• Avoid using hair products that contain too many chemicals them.

Do not wear your hair with tight hairstyles that can lead to breakage of hair and eventually lead to loss of hair.

• Keep your scalp and hair as clean as you can.

Healthy Diet to maintain healthy hair

Foods that can help prevent hair Loss

We've discussed how crucial it is to eat healthy and balanced diet to stop and treat hair loss. A few of the foods that can be extremely beneficial in preventing loss of hair include the following.

Beans - Beans can be a excellent source of Vitamin C, B vitamin protein , and other important minerals that are extremely beneficial to ensure optimal growth of hair. Additionally, they contain a substantial amount of iron , which is another vital nutrient that helps in the prevention of hair loss.

Salmon - This specific type of fish that is fatty is an absolute gem in the fight against hair loss. In addition to containing a substantial amount of protein as well as B vitamins Salmon is also believed to be a abundant source of omega-3 fatty acids that play a crucial role in encouraging healthy hair growth.

Eggs - This easy food isn't quite as easy as it might seem in terms of the nutrients it provides. Eggs are a great source of protein, as well as other minerals, like sulfur. They also contain iron, which is extremely efficient in carrying oxygen to hair follicles.

These are just a few of the many food items that can assist you prevent loss of hair. Incorporating healthy food items like these into your diet is easy and simultaneously an extremely beneficial favor you can perform for your body. Give your body the best treatment as your body will be grateful to you.

Chapter 21: Natural Herbs For Healthy Hair

When you reach 45 or more males and females are more susceptible to losing hair. Males suffer from baldness, while women experience hair that is thin. If your hair starts falling out on a regular basis, it could affect your self-confidence and self-esteem. The good news is that aside from the solutions discussed previously there are also some natural herbs that can be used to keep your hair from falling out or stopping it.

When you are using this herb, also known as "saw palmetto" this herb can assist in the prevention of hair loss since it inhibits the growth of dihydrotestosterone (DHT) within your body. This herb is available in extract or tincture form. It's also a component in many shampoos. Some people use it internally to increase the advantages. Saw palmetto helps restore balance to the scalp as it cleanses pores and encourages healthy circulation of blood.

Another herb that can help promote good hair health is rosemary. It is rich in antioxidants that help restore balance to your scalp. It can be combined with almond oil and massaged onto your scalp to stop hair loss and hair loss. It is also possible to apply rosemary to your hair to rinse your hair after you've finished shampooing. Add two teaspoons fresh rosemary into the glass or crystal pitcher. In the same pitcher, add one cup of boiling water, and allow it to steep for 20 minutes. The herb should be strained out, and mix in the vinegar in a tablespoon. Apply the mixture to your hair following washed it. Don't rinse your hair immediately afterward.

It is also possible to take the essential herb Pygeum, which is similar as saw palmetto. The herb is commonly combined with saw palmetto to stop prostate enlargement. Other herbs that aid in thin hair and baldness are the nettle root and pygeum Africanum.

It is common to find horsetail in shampoos to help to treat hair. The Horsetail herb has a high amount of silica. It is beneficial for skin and hair health. It is also ingested but be cautious and limit your intake to the limits for consumption. The most potent formula of the herbal remedy is as a pill which is dried by freezing. If you are using it to treat hair loss it is best to drink it in tea form. Simply add one tablespoon of crushed horsehair plant to 1 cup water. It is also possible to include sugar or honey to make tea more tasty and sweet. This herb can correct hormonal imbalances that lead to hair loss.

In the event that your hair has begun to thin because of hormonal imbalances due to menopausal changes or pregnancy It is possible to treat it with the herbal remedies nettle and corn silk. They can reverse the effects of these imbalances.

When your hair starts thin due to problems with your adrenal glands it is possible to treat this issue by taking herbs like astragalas and the licorice. Women can also use estrogen-based supplements to combat the issues with hair loss. If you have a severe medical condition or are pregnant, you should avoid taking the licorice.

There are also herbal supplements to treat hair loss that can be beneficial for the body. These include he shou wu fo-ti, yucca and fo ti. they can ease anxiety, for instance the stress that is linked to loss of hair.

Chapter 22: The Genetic Connection

Many have believed that baldness was something that is genetic. As you've read in the preceding chapter, this is not entirely true. There are different types of hair loss disorders which are hereditary.

Experts believe that they have finally identified the gene that could be responsible for the alopecia areata condition. According to the most recent studies, the gene is associated with a variety of auto-immune conditions that include type 1 diabetes as well as Rheumatoid arthritis.

The gene known as ULBP3 that is not supposed to be present in hair follicles, was discovered in the hair cells of those suffering with Alopecia areata. The reason this gene is harmful to hair cells is because it is a magnet for cytotoxic cells which are immune cells which aids the body in fighting disease and destroy damaged cells. But, ULBP3 will start attacking healthy cells even if it isn't able to detect any injury or damage.

Another aspect that ULBP3 will draw is NKG2D cells that are known as receptors for killing. NKG2D has been linked to other autoimmune diseases, and this is the biomarker that is used to determine this genetic hair loss issue Alopecia areata, also known as alopecia rhinitis.

What is this referring to?

It was found that the two the genes ULBP3 as well as NKG2D share a common function in the organs they are found in and are located together in the follicles of people with genetic baldness, researchers were able examine their behaviour and finally identified an underlying pattern.

The pattern, or pathway that they found is always a similar way: ULBP3 reacts when the NKG2D gene has sent the signal of warning--which is the gene for killing--to the ULBP3 gene, triggering the process of killing the surrounding cells. The discovery of this has led researchers to develop potential treatments that include interception of these gene that is causing problems.

Conclusion

A lot of people are opting for homemade cosmetics and health products as they're realizing the advantages of using organic, natural ingredients. Products purchased from the store appear and can smell fantastic but they're stuffed with chemicals and toxic substances that could have harmful effects on our body.

In the process of making and using home-made natural beauty and health products We are confident that what is put into these products is not going to harm or cause harm to us. We are in control of the products we put on our bodies. We are able to take care of our body and hair with the use of all natural ingredients and create the perfect scents for the times we require it.

In addition, homemade shampoos are simple to make. If you've ran out of the usual shampoos, then all you have to do is go into the kitchen to create a batch of the items you typically have in your home.

Hair treatments and shampoos made from home are fun, easy to make and cost-effective and it's due to this that millions of people are turning to these types of products.

www.ingramcontent.com/pod-product-compliance
Lightning Source LLC
Chambersburg PA
CBHW060328030426
42336CB00011B/1255